VESSEL

Writing Through the Fears of Death, Responsibility, Isolation, and Meaninglessness

Dr. Nancy Farber Kent

VESSEL
Writing Through the Fears of Death, Responsibility,
Isolation, and Meaninglessness
Copyright © Kalliope Pearl Publishing 2020

ISBN: 978-1-7348851-1-8

Cover design: Eli Lynn
Editorial team: Colleen Nolan Murphy, Lisa Plotkin, Mark Salzberg
Music recording team: Nancy Farber Kent, Gabrielle Giarratano,
Nick Kochaneck, Josh Tindall

Death

Responsibility

Isolation

Meaninglessness

… THE 4 GIVENS OF EXISTENCE

(YALOM, 1980)

INTRODUCTION

Dear Reader,

Welcome to Vessel. Thank you for taking the time to read this book.

My hope is to be a model, and through modeling of my own process, you may learn something about

1. The givens of existence we all face: **death, responsibility, isolation, meaninglessness.**
2. The process of writing-as-therapy.
3. The process of Gestalt therapy and how dialoguing with parts of self and imaginary others can help to resolve inner conflicts.
4. The reality that we all have "voices" inside our head.
5. The reality that whatever you are feeling, millions of others are feeling the same thing at any given moment.
6. The reality that you are **never alone.**

This book was written in real time as a series of psychotherapy "sessions" with my therapist-self. I invite you to join me as I engage in writing-as-therapy, Gestalt two-chair "dialogues" with self and others, and examining the "givens of existence" as I work toward my goal of achieving **"one song on the radio before I die."**

My hope is that you will learn something and relate as you join me on my current adventure and on my reflections back on my travels through addiction, suicidality, and being the psychologist-on-the-other-side.

You may be a fellow psychotherapist. You may be a student-of-psychotherapy. You may be a fellow human being traveling along your own life journey. Whatever your motivation for reading this book, I hope you enjoy it and learn something that will be helpful to you.

So, sit back, lie down, or cuddle up with your Kindle.

"Come along my journey, for it's your journey. I will be your vessel. You can be mine."

- *A link to a live recording of the song "Vessel" is included at the end of this book.*

PROLOGUE

It's May. It's 1987.

Congratulations, Nancy. You graduated from college. Hooray!

My mother is so happy. She's so happy that she made it to the graduation despite the last year of chemotherapy and radiation and losing her beautiful, red hair. She is happy that she is still alive and that she gets to see her baby graduate college.

Of course, it doesn't really mean that much to me. Because I'm confused about my life. Where is it going? Everybody else seems to have jobs and careers and how-to-have-a-boyfriend figured out. I don't know what I'm doing.

So, I decide to follow my brother to Atlanta, Georgia where he's working. He lets me move in with him while I figure it out.

I get my first job. I'm doing singing telegrams. It's a good way to learn my way around Atlanta because I have to read the map to figure out where I'm going every time I get a call for a job.

I just got a call that they want me to go to a hospital and sing the "Get Well Song" for a little girl who is a patient there. This should be fun.

I put on my standard singing telegram costume they've given me of fish net stockings, a leotard and a hot pink blazer. I feel a little funny wearing this to the hospital, but this is the costume they've given me so here I go.

I arrive. The hospital staff directs me to the children's ward. They direct me to the children's cancer ward. Suddenly, I realize as I'm talking to this little girl and learning about her situation, that I am confronted with a child who may not leave this hospital. She's probably not going to get better. She's going to die. Soon.

I stand there, kind of frozen. Am I going to sing the "Get Well Song?" Holy shit. I *can't* sing the "Get Well Song." What the hell am I going to do?

I improvise. *"Hey, so tell me. What's your favorite band?"* I ask. *Do you have a favorite band?"*

"I love Duran Duran," she says.

Okay. I decide to improvise and sing a Duran Duran song :

I dance around like a goofball and sing, *"Her name is Rio and she dances on the sand! Just like that river twisting through a dusty land…"*

I sing Duran Duran. She joins in with me. We laugh. We have fun.

Whew! Made it. Somehow. Got through that one. Improvised. Improvisation. Improvised.

So where is this going? Where am I going now? What is going to happen with my career? Am I going to continue along the path of singing? Am I going to keep looking for a "real job" and work my way into the Human Resources field which is what I am hoping to do at this time?

I do like helping people and I've always been an observer of human behavior. I've always wanted to be a psychologist. I know my mother doesn't think it's a great idea because she would prefer I did something more glamorous. But I know, deep down, she will support any decision I make. She encourages me to study for my GRE and go back to graduate school.

In the meantime, as I'm studying for my GRE, I decide to find a job in Human Resources.

I apply for a job as a Personnel Assistant. They ask if I would be interested in a job as an "Inventory Field Trainer." I get to travel around the Southeast and train people in how to keep their inventory for office supplies. I know nothing about office supplies or inventory but I will learn. Cool! I get to travel around and stay in hotels and meet people and count boxes.

I can sense that some of the managers like me, respect and appreciate me. I can sense that some of the managers don't like a strong woman making her way in the old boys' network. One of the managers makes comments about my breasts. It's 1987. I've never heard of sexual harassment. I just know that I don't feel like I'm going to make it in this company. I decide to quit.

"Don't quit your job until you have another job!" my father admonishes. Fear. Security. Fear.

But I quit anyway. And I quickly find a job waitressing. I'm a terrible waitress. I spill things on the customers and when people order wine I say, "Your wine waitress will be with you in a moment," and then run back to the kitchen and beg someone to go open up a bottle of wine for me because I just can't seem to master the technique of unscrewing a cork.

I waitress for a few months and then find a part time job working as an administrative assistant for architects. I get to type up specs and learn about architecture. It's interesting. I share a desk with Ellen, the business manager. **"Would you like a butterscotch?"** she offers me as I'm typing. It's a little thing but a big thing to me because it's a warm gesture and it makes me feel like I belong. I sing Karen Carpenter songs as I type and Tom and Markham, the architects, laugh. I can sing and be myself. It feels good.

I know it's temporary, though, because I'm feeling the internal and external pressure to find a full-time job that somehow fits with my degree. I want so badly to prove to my mother that I can be successful. I want to be happy and not feel like such a loser. I want to not be so depressed.

"NANCY, I CAN'T BE THERE FOR YOU THE WAY I USED TO BE. YOU'RE GOING TO HAVE TO FIGURE THINGS OUT FOR YOURSELF," my mother tells me over the phone after her cancer comes back and she is sick and no longer capable of being the one who can give me advice and get me out of my emotional turmoil.

Okay. I'll figure it out. I'll just keep applying for jobs. Letters. Phone calls. Follow up phone calls. Rejection. Rejection. Rejection. Why can't I find a job? Why isn't anyone interested? Come on! I've got to get on my feet and show my mother I will be okay before she dies. Before she dies. Why isn't this working?

I don't know now that this may be a sign. That sometimes when you're fighting so hard to make something go a certain way, it means that there's another way you're supposed to go…

Home. I'm supposed to go home. I'm supposed to go back to New York and be with my mother while there is still time.

Am I going to be able to figure it out, figure out my career path and what I'm supposed to do? Am I ever going to find a boyfriend and stop feeling like there's something wrong with me?

And how do I do this while my mother is back in New York with cancer herself? I don't know how long she has to live. **FEAR OF DEATH**

"Nan, you need to get out of there. You need to go home and be with your mother," my friend Holly tells me.

You're right, Holly. I need to go home and be with my mother. Because her time, *her time*, is limited. The rest will be on hold. I'll figure out my career. I'll figure out what I'm supposed to do and where I'm supposed to go. It will happen. I'll figure out why I often feel like the loneliest person on the planet. I'll figure out the meaning of my life. It will happen.

All the questions will be answered in time. I don't know any of this now, of course. But I will ... one day....

It's May. It's 2017.

Congratulations, Nancy. You graduated from college. Hooray!

My mother is so happy. She's so happy for so many reasons. My mother, a self-deprecating gifted pianist, always encouraged my music. She was so proud of me when I sang and wrote songs.

I would get up on stage and perform for her as a child and as an adolescent, but secretly I preferred locking myself up in my room with my four- track recorder and mixing harmonies that no one would hear. And, yet, I must admit, secretly, there was always a part of me that wanted to share my recordings.

But a real musician? Could I take myself seriously as a musician? I could not read music. Neither could my mother. She played piano by ear. Everything in the key of C.

I always felt somewhat embarrassed when I tried to collaborate with other musicians. Yes, I could sing. Yes, I had a good ear. And yes, I had learned some guitar. But what is a dominant seventh chord? And how do I communicate with other musicians when I don't know the language? And how is it that some people know how to read rhythm through notes?

I longed to be "real" musician. I longed to learn the language I could not speak, nor read, nor write.

So, when James decided to go back to school for medicine, I decided that this would be a good time for me to go back to school as well.

It was a gradual process. It started with mustering up the courage to just say out loud, *"I want to go back to school for music."* There. It's out there in the universe. It exists now.
Before I met James, I conducted a couple of informational interviews with directors of music programs. Is it possible? What courses would I need to take? Can I find a way to do this while still working as a psychologist? I remember this one program director hearing the fear and self-doubt in my voice and telling me this was my "Come to Jesus moment." Hmmm....

Small steps. My roommate, Bonnie, encouraged me to start with one course. So, I took an online Music Theory class through a local community college. I loved it! I fell in love with Music Theory. Yes...I could do this. I wanted to do this. *I would do this.*

So ... how to do this....

James was interviewing for medical school. I was working at the State Psychiatric Hospital. I decided to take piano lessons. Group piano lessons at the Community Music School. I hesitantly shared with my piano teacher, Andrew, that I wanted to go back to school and study music. *There it is again. It's real. I've said it out loud.*

Audition. I need to prepare for an audition. Andrew guided me to Joe, a voice teacher. Joe helped me prepare two opera pieces (Me? Singing opera? Really?!) Joe believed in me: **"You have more high notes in there than you realize."** Hmmm ... And here I thought I was limited to my Alto range, which for some reason, I always felt like being an Alto meant I was second class. Maybe because Altos are rarely given the melody in choirs.

My friend, Val, and I took a drive out to see the town where James would be going to Medical School and to just take a peek at a college in a neighboring town that had a music program: Lebanon Valley College.

At first, I was afraid of the change. "There's not enough mountains out here!" I freaked out the in car. "I won't feel okay living here!" Not enough mountains, I feared. The unknown. FEAR. Fear that I would not be able to feel like myself. That a part of myself would cease to exist. **FEAR OF ISOLATION.** INTRAPERSONAL ISOLATION.

But then we stopped at LVC. I bumped into Mr. Strohman, the brass teacher. "Is it possible?" I asked him. "**Of course, it is,**" he smiled. I drove back home and called the director of the program, Dr. Mecham. "Is it possible?" I asked him. "**WHY NOT?**" he responded.

Anything is possible. *"It's never too late to be what you might have been,"* says George Eliot.

So, I completed my application, prepared (for my audition), and drove back out to Annville, PA for an audition. Dr. Lister, who was to become my vocal mentor and friend, listened to me sing. Dr. Morell tested my ear. Dr. Mecham interviewed me. I left feeling so excited. *I'm doing this! I'm really doing this!* And a few days later, I received my acceptance letter in the mail. Hooray!

We moved to Hershey a few months later and I began my music program in the Fall. The first week of class I had a total panic attack. I can't do this! The other kids already know so much more about music theory. They've been formally studying music their whole lives. I'm behind! I'm a menopausal freshman! What am I doing? But Dr. Morell and Dr. Lovell offered me extra help and I caught up. And then I started to do really well. *Hey, I get this … I love this …*

So, it's been an amazing three years, filled with many new challenges. I have learned so much. I completed a goal. And that feels great. I've learned how to collaborate and communicate with other musicians. And that feels really great. I know the language. I'm a certified, stamped, degreed "musician." Still insecure, but a lot more confident than before, for sure.

So ... where is this going? Where am I going now? What is going to happen with my career?

Am I going to continue my work as a psychologist? Am I going to compose more? Am I going to do both? Where is this all leading to now?

One song on the radio before I die.

There. I've said it. I've said it out loud. It exists.

I guess deep down I would like to have **one song on the radio before I die.** Leave my legacy. I don't have human children. I have songs. So, if I can put one out there to carry on, then somehow my life has meaning?

FEAR OF MEANINGLESSNESS.

Would I like to have more than **one song on the radio before I die?** Perhaps. I'm not sure. Reservations. Fears. Fears of being consumed and feeling the pressure that I see a lot of musicians feel. If it becomes pressure, and I lose the joy, then it has lost its purpose. Then again, any work or passion can be approached with pressure rather than joy.

Would I like to put closure on my work as a psychologist and identify only as a musician? Perhaps. I'm not sure. I do believe there is a divine plan for me and things that I am called to do to play my part in helping the world. So, some of my work as a psychologist may be necessary for me to fulfill a higher purpose—but then again, even when I worked at the state hospital, that thing that I did that seemed to benefit the patients most was the music. Hmmm....

I guess I do want to move toward the merge of music/psychology that I'd been experimenting with in the state hospital. It was all integrated there. Right now, though, my plate is filled with individual and couple clients. I am not in a place where I can just uproot that.

Hmmm ... Maybe it's okay that for right now, I don't know where it's all going.

Maybe it even helps right now to just write about goals and know that *when I write, things come into fruition.*

Okay, it's 7:08 am. Time to go eat breakfast, walk the dogs, and head into the office, serenely, presently, with joy, openness, and faith.

SESSION #2

....

Perhaps if I approach my writing as process/progress notes, the goal will come to fruition as it does with clients. Of course, with clients as well, the goals change. With more self-awareness, goals do sometimes change.

One song on the radio before I die: This has been a goal most of my life, as was finding the man with whom I could live happily ever after (more important to me—so this is probably why I achieved this first—finally—happily married at 50 ... worth waiting for).

I digress. But I want to digress. Just like my clients—I have something else that came up that I need to focus on today. It's related to my goal, I guess.

James and I were asked to share a blurb for Graduation Sunday at church. Be acknowledged with a photo, mention our degrees, our plans for the future.

Keep the focus on him graduating from Medical School is what I wanted. I don't want to have my graduation announced at church. My recital was my graduation. It was my celebration of "I can do this. I can compose not only by ear but I can put it down on paper so other musicians can read and play it. I can gather a group of musicians together and watch them translate what I wrote into music." That was my graduation.

No, I don't want my graduation celebrated at church.

HER: How come?

ME: How come?

HER: Yes. How come you don't want your graduation celebrated at church?

ME: I don't know. I guess I don't want to draw the attention to myself. Because if I do, I might feel pressure. I guess I'm afraid that if people know I completed my degree in music, there might be more expectations of me? I mean, James says I should be flattered when people ask me to join different musical groups. But it's hard sometimes because obviously, I can't do everything, and I have to do things I feel called to do, but then you have to say "no" and disappoint people.

HER: So ... you don't want to disappoint.

ME: Well, of course not. I don't want to disappoint. But at the same time. I don't want to disappoint myself either by running around in circles saying "yes," to everything, even if they are things that I don't feel called to do.

I remember when I drove across the country and people I would meet would say things like, "Oh, if you're going here, you should go see THIS monument, or THAT park, or THAT museum ... do THIS, do THAT, don't miss THIS or THAT...

Noooooo!

No. No. No. People on my journey, I know you mean well, and you just want to me to experience something that was so wonderful for you, but you see, there's only so much time, and I have to have my own experience. I have to listen to my intuition and see where it guides me. It may be to a different place than you were guided.

HER: There you go....

ME: What do you mean?

HER: I mean, when people ask you to do things you don't feel called to do, you just tell them that.

ME: Doesn't that sound a little haughty and self-righteous?

HER: Well, maybe just keep the focus on the things you do feel called to do. And give all your enthusiasm and passion to those things. And just be gracious and grateful when you set the boundary and say "no" to the other things.

ME: I guess that makes sense. I just don't want to seem selfish.

HER: Do you think doing what you feel called to do is selfish?

ME: No.

HER: Okay then. So why don't you meditate on the idea of being included in the graduation program...

ME: Sounds good.

Thanks for listening....

SESSION #2 (ADDENDUM)

Well, as it turned out, I allowed myself to be included in the Graduation Program.

Because when I was told "We really like to celebrate people's achievements," I realized that it is an achievement to be celebrated, and people at church like to share in each other's joys. And I should be grateful that there are people who want to share in my joy. Perhaps, also, it inspires others to see that they too, can achieve goals and dreams at any age. It's not just about me. It's about everyone. So, when I thought about it, I realized that not allowing myself to be included in the program, *that* would be selfish.

Anyhow, regarding my fear of expectations, it's up to me to set boundaries when I'm asked to do things I don't feel called to do.

FEAR OF RESPONSIBILITY.

I make choices. It's up to me.

Like my private practice. After hitting a point of stress overload, anger, resentment and taking it all out on James, I came to the realization that I really want to move away from individual psychotherapy and toward the merge of music-psychotherapy-dementia groups that I was experimenting with at the psychiatric hospital. I know I'm being called to this.

"Follow your dream, Dr. Farber!" said one of the patients in
the hospital when I told my ward I was leaving to go back to
school for music. There are lots of ways to be helpful. And
there are lots of people out there, both old and new in the
counseling field who are eager and excited to do individual
therapy. Trust this work to them. Allow myself to walk toward
the projects that call me now....

So, James assures me it is okay to start letting go and moving
toward the next thing. That it is okay not to take on too many
new individual clients. For this is the only way to free up the
space to create what I long to create. But of course, all the fear
and self-doubt come in:

*REALLY, NANCY, YOU'RE GOING TO TURN AWAY
INDIVIDUAL CLIENTS? HOW SELFISH OF YOU!*

*REALLY, NANCY, YOU ARE GOING TO TURN
AWAY INDIVIDUAL CLIENTS? THAT'S MONEY YOU
WON'T BE EARNING. WILL YOU HAVE ENOUGH
TO PAY THE BILLS AS YOU WORK ON
TRANSITIONING?*

My dear self:

*I know you are full of fear. We all are afraid to "take the leap" toward
our heart's desires. Yet remember when you were afraid to take the leap
into private practice. You so feared going out on your own. And look!
You've done it. You can do anything you set your mind to. And you
WILL be helping people. Perhaps even more people if you're doing groups.
As far as money goes, trust the process. Do what you love.... One day at a
time. Do you have food today, Nancy? Yes. A bed to sleep in today,
Nancy? Yes.*

All my needs are met today. Trust the process. All will be
well...

SESSION #3

....

ME: Hello Dr. Farber. How are you this morning?

HER: Well, Nancy. How are you?

ME: Good. I just meditated. And it helps me to feel more centered. I've started meditating 5 minutes a day. My brain is slowing down in a good way. I'm starting to be in the moment more and not What-If-ing it as much.

HER: Good. How can I help you today?

ME: Well, I had a realization this morning while I was walking the dogs. I read a text that a friend had sent that said that enlightenment is when we no longer worry and when we see those mystical coincidences more and more. I want that. I want to worry less. Then suddenly I thought about piano and I how I want to get better at it and how I was planning to take lessons through the Community Music School this fall because it costs less and then reflecting that I really want to continue to take lessons as an enrolled student even though it costs a little more because I want to be accountable and I want to take myself seriously as a musician. It may sound silly but there is something about continuing to be an enrolled music student, taking the class for credit, and having to be evaluated at the end of the semester that helps to motivate me to work harder and achieve my goal. I suck at playing piano but I believe that with practice I can get better. I mean I've managed to become a "good enough" guitar player to be respected for being able to play and sing. I've practiced. But piano---piano intimidates me. But I believe I can do it.

So, what I'm saying is if I let go of financial fears and allow myself to move forward as an enrolled student who will be earning a grade, it will help me. Does this make sense?

HER: It sounds like you know what is right for you.

ME: Well, yes. I do. But there is still that guilt that creeps in. That "how dare you" voice.

HER: How dare you....

ME: Yes. Well, Dr. Farber. I've got to go. I've got to let you go. You have clients awaiting.

HER: Yes, we will talk more. Just know this ---I love you!

ME: I love you too! ☺

SESSION #4

....

Thanks for agreeing to meet with me, self. For allowing me to take the time for some writing therapy. Because writing is what leads me to my truth. Self-therapy. *"Writing down the bones"* as Natalie Goldberg phrased it.

I look at the clock on my computer: I see that it's 12:44 and I worry about having enough time—I plan backwards: new client at 3:15, want to get to the office by 2:45, leave here by 2:30 – that gives me one hour and 45 minutes from now to dry my hair, get dressed, eat lunch—do I have time for a 45-minute session (max) with myself? Yes, I do. Thank you.

Whew! I knew I needed a session today because my head was racing all morning. I got hit by generalized anxiety, and then later by anger when I resented a friend who was making demands on me.

But it's up to me to set the boundary. Boundaries. Boundaries. They're hard because I still feel guilty—like it's my job to solve everybody else's problems. But I need to trust that when I feel called to help in a situation—I help. It feels natural and there is joy in it. I tend to want to help people more when they don't ask for help—when they expect nothing. The downtrodden. The outcasts. But when people push me and make demands on me—that just makes me want to run away. Is that bad? Is that selfish?

HER: What do you think?

ME: I think I'm conflicted. I don't like the feeling of helping someone when they are ungrateful, or when they see my helping them as an invitation to keep demanding more and more. I've done this before.

And I've also been the person who did this to others when I was so screwed up. I don't want to be that person; nor do I want to get into that dance with others who behave that way. For me, if someone just ignored me when I was like that, I eventually stopped making demands on them. I would find someone else to bug. Until I learned how to take responsibility for myself. So, I feel the best course of action is to do the same: ignore. But there is still guilt there.

Yet, when I focus my efforts on the helpful things that I want to do, that I feel called to do, like I'm so excited that I ordered a used WAIS on E-bay, and I'm going to use it to do some pre-testing/post-testing with my stroke client to see how music theory lessons as cognitive stimulation affect his processing speed and perhaps memory; as I focus my efforts in this direction, and I'm so excited because I also ordered a music theory workbook and will begin developing my "program," not only does the guilt lift, but so does the anger. Because now I am focusing on helping in the way I feel called, and I'm helping someone who is downtrodden, who does not make demands, and who is grateful.

I mean we're all capable of being grateful and polite. No matter how mentally ill we may be. We all have the capacity to have good manners.

HER: *So, it sounds like you're not so keen about putting your "helping" efforts out to those without good manners.*

ME: Well, even when I worked in the psychiatric hospital, this one client, let's call him "Wayne" for fun. Well, he would get psychotic and flip out and I would stay with him and remain calm. But he didn't expect anything. And when I stayed with him, and helped him calm down, he thanked me with his eyes. Actually, most of the patients were that way. They would flip out. But they were also the truly downtrodden. And they appreciated when you were there for them.

HER: You use the word downtrodden a lot.

ME: Yes, because that's how I see the ones that I'm drawn to help. Now this friend of mine, the one who makes demands, maybe it's someone else's calling to intervene with her. I mean I believe we are all like pieces of a puzzle and we find where we fit. Relationships. Find the ones that fit. It took me a long time to find the person whose puzzle piece fit in perfectly with mine. Maybe that's how it is in all relationships. So, I suppose if I trust my gut feelings, I will know who I'm supposed to help, or befriend, or marry as I did. ☺

HER: Smiley face?

ME: Indeed, because I just had a therapeutic breakthrough that made me smile. Thank you for listening.

HER: No problem. I feel called to help you! After all, I'm you. ☺

ME: Yes, and look at that. It's only 1:07. Not even 20 minutes of our time. Off to go finish the hair and eat leftovers.

SESSION #5

....

One song on the radio before I die. After that will I live happily ever after? No. There is no final endpoint. Cinderella must continue on and work out the kinks in her relationship with Prince Charming for her entire life and enjoy the ups and downs because that is life.

It is a goal though. And working towards a goal gives me a sense of purpose. **FEAR OF MEANINGLESSNESS**

Let's review existential theory (Yalom) – **death, responsibility, isolation, meaninglessness** - and remind ourselves that every day we may encounter some masked form of the fears that accompany the givens of existence.

So, having a goal, having a purpose—this keeps fear of meaninglessness at bay.

But **FEAR OF ISOLATION**. Oh, that old fear of isolation.

So, I can be surrounded by people as I was all day yesterday and still feel isolated. Still feel lonely.

Because I need to feel understood. Need to feel that I exist.

So, when I'm visiting the church where James grew up, where I'm culturally "different," where I feel like an appendage rather than a full human being, it happens so gradually that I don't even notice it but somewhere along the way I realize that I am disappearing. I'm polite. I'm friendly. "How are you? Nice to see you." But I am really just being a polite machine making the best of being in a situation where I sense that my true self would not be welcomed.

If she were, she would do something like fly up on the alter, say, "Okay, men, let me help you out with this ministry stuff," share my philosophy that I believe G-d wants us to dance and sing and be joyous—put on a little disco—"*Everybody Dance Now!*"—and get the people moving, dancing, laughing. I would know that G-d was smiling down (G-d who for me is genderless), happy that his/her/it's/their people were enjoying life. Men and women and animals and gays and straights and blacks and whites and Christians and Muslims and Hindus and Buddhists and Jews and transgendered and rich and poor and short and tall and plants and bees and everything else living or not-living according to human perceptions would be dancing together.

Whew! I went on and on there. And now I feel better. I feel connected to everyone and everything. Sometimes it helps to just write about it - to express it - to my imaginary audience whom one day will be my circle. *I will be your vessel. You can be mine.*

Yay! **FEAR OF ISOLATION** is now at bay.

I exist.

Off to walk the dogs, play piano, and prepare the WAIS for pre-testing with my client.

Thanks for listening…

SESSION NOTE ADDENDUM: I *will* go to the Friends of Jazz gathering tonight. Yes, I am afraid. But my philosophy has always been if it both scares AND excites you, then it's something you should do. It's okay if I haven't had time to put my "book" together perfectly and professionally. A few lead sheets in a folder will be fine. No pressure. I will sit back and enjoy and watch and learn and sing a song or two...

SESSION ADDENDUM FOLLOW UP NOTE:

I did it! I did it! I did it! And now I am on a natural high today.

I almost didn't go. I almost let fear take over... "Maybe I'll wait and go next month."

"You'll be mad at yourself if you don't go," James said. **"You'll feel good after you've gone."**

You're right, cheerleader. Thank you.

So, I went. I sat down in the front row and put my folder with lead sheets on the table. Andy, the evening's leader came around to see who would be sitting in this evening. *"Horn players? Drummers? Pianists?"* He looked at me inquisitively.

"I'm a vocalist," I said confidently.

"Don't use the word singer, my jazz teacher, Tim, had taught me. Vocalist is the professional term.

Andy told me he'd bring me up after a couple of instrumentals. *"Do you know what you want to sing?"* he asked.

"Yes, *Skylark* and *Honeysuckle Rose.* And I brought lead sheets if that helps."

"Oh, great. That makes it a lot easier," he said. Tim had taught me to be prepared with my lead sheets. I had asked Tim one time why some instrumentalists seemed not to like having vocalists join them. He told me it's all about doing your homework and being prepared. I can't waltz in like a diva expecting others to figure out what I want to sing and how to play it. I must be a fellow musician. Doing my homework. Having my chord charts. Understanding music theory. Knowing how to communicate with other musicians.

I sang my two songs and communicated well. I was more nervous about "communicating" than I was about singing. But I looked and I listened. I followed when Andy cued me to go to the B section. I enjoyed listening to the solos on the trumpet and the saxophone. I got excited when Andy said, *"Okay, now just vocals and drums on the A section"* ---so much fun—I could experiment with vocal triple lutzes with just a driving drumbeat behind me---yay!

I sat back down feeling good and satisfied---I did it—I communicated. I sang well. Now I could just enjoy watching everyone else.

Watching and listening to everyone else. Yes, this is great!

Watching and listening to everyone else. Yes, I'm feeling it. I'm in the zone. ☺

Watching and listening to everyone else. Hey, that saxophonist is back up there. Hmmm…

Watching and listening to everyone else. That piano player came back up for a second time too.

Watching and listening to everyone else. And the trumpet player is back as well. Well, I think they know him. He's probably an old friend. Be patient, Nancy. Don't push yourself. They don't know you yet.

But they don't know the saxophone or piano player either. They are both new. And they're a lot younger than you. How come they get to go back up? Is it the boys club again?

Be patient.

I decide to stand up and walk around. When suddenly, a man with a saxophone and lots of wild energy comes over and introduces himself—Joe—Old Joe. Starts to tell me he's played with these guys lots—maybe he'll go join them on a song. Okay, I'll hang out and watch Old Joe play a tune. I'll stay until the end. Maybe next time I'll get to do more.

Old Joe gets up and joins them and then Andy says, *"Okay we're going to do one last tune"* and invites all the horn players up to join. Suddenly, I notice that just about everybody is back up on stage. Not me. They're just improvising. Trading 4s or 8s. Hey, wait a minute. I can do this too. I can get up and improvise. Can't I be an instrument too? Please let me. Please let me.

I wander over to Old Joe and ask him if he thinks Andy would mind if I got up and grabbed the mic and did some improvising as well. "Get up there!!" Old Joe encourages me.

I leap up on stage, grab the mic, and to my surprise, Andy is happy that I joined them. He looks at me and cues me that I will get the next solo.

I improvise. I vocalize. I sing high, low, up, down, all around—triple salchow. I let the music move through me. Andy starts blowing a note on this instrument that I don't even know what it is—some piano you blow into—and then the sax and piano player join in with the same note on the same rhythm, and then I join in with a harmony on the same rhythm and we are making music and we are communicating and I am in heaven!!

FEAR OF RESPONSIBILITY

That is the existential fear that needed to be overcome in this moment. I had a choice. Sit back. Be a victim. Assume they don't want me there.

OR make a choice. Is it okay? Yes, it's okay. Then go do it. Did it. And as I join the fellow musicians, I find that I belong.

ISOLATION at bay as well.

Thanks for listening.

SESSION #6

....

Good morning. And welcome to Session #6. I think weekly sessions will be helpful. Once a week, same day every week. Structure helps me to stay focused on my goal:

One Song on the Radio Before I Die

I wonder about my goal—the timing. Am I avoiding by saying "before I die?" Should I move it up and give it a time limit? 5 years? 2 years? Why do I say "before I die?"

HER: What do you think?

ME: I think I'm afraid to take myself too seriously. I also think I experience guilt for wanting to pursue my dream. I fear being "self-indulgent." I think that I am also aware of competing demands and other things that are important and want to allow myself the space to be able to fulfill the other roles that I feel called to fill—good psychologist, good wife.

I think I've watched "It's A Wonderful Life," way too many times and remember how George Bailey always wanted to make it to Europe but never did because he was helping other people, and in the end when he was suicidal, he realized, like my mother taught me, that the only thing that truly matters in life is that you're surrounded by people who really love you. So, I guess I feel like I want to give myself an out, that if it never happens, it's okay, because I have what matters most—love.

HER: What happened to George Bailey after the crisis? What happened after?

ME: I don't know. The movie ends there.

HER: *Do you think he eventually made it to Europe?*

ME: I don't know. Perhaps he did. I see where you're going with this.

HER: *Tell me.*

ME: He has his suicidal crisis. He saved the bank. He saved himself. Perhaps after he experienced his own dark night of the soul his life carried on and he said—Okay, now it's time to follow my dream. Perhaps after all the kids went to college, George and Mary took off to Europe. We don't know. I've had my suicidal crisis too. I made it through the dark night of the soul.

HER: *So now what?*

ME: So now it's okay to follow my dreams…I guess I just still have trouble with guilt—I still hear that little voice, that "lower power" saying, "How dare you do what you want to do!!" Ugh. The Devil.

I guess I still fear it's selfish. But it's not selfish. I know music helps others as well. Music heals as well. Like just this morning. I'm walking the dogs and I feel myself experiencing a little bit of the darkness for no particular reason, and then my Leonard Bernstein CD starts playing the medley from West Side Story and I feel myself smile and my step becomes lighter as I sing "I like to be in America…okay by me in America…." and I'm lifted. Thank you, Leonard Bernstein. Thank you for helping lift my spirit. Perhaps I can do the same.

HER: *Small font.*

ME: Small voice. I'd like to make it bigger. Just don't want it to become too big---arrogant. Been to that extreme too. Want to stay middle.

HER: *Okay, so it sounds like you're starting to see that it's okay to want to follow your dreams. And that your dreams are not completely self-indulgent. That music is a way of helping others as well. And that you've been to the darkest place one can go. You've been to the point of wanting to die. And now you're not. So maybe George Bailey eventually did do something he's always dreamed of doing. We don't know. But regardless, maybe it's okay if Nancy does.*

ME: Maybe.

HER: *You're wondering about the timeline though.*

ME: Yes, because I know with therapy, it helps to have time limits. If we know we have a limited number of sessions, it helps us to focus on reaching the goal. If I have a deadline for anything, I work to meet that deadline. So, okay. I can do this. I'm just wondering about the deadline. But I don't want to decide that today. I'm not ready to decide if I want to make the deadline sooner than "before I die."

HER: *That's okay. You're making progress.*

ME: Thank you Dr. Self.

HER: *You're welcome. See you next week....*

SESSION #7

....

One song on the radio before I die.

Before I die.

FEAR OF DEATH – The 4th existential fear.

Not actual death. Not death of my body. I have had enough mystical coincidences in my life to assure me that all will be well when I cross over (of course check with me again, when I'm at that point. I may be scared!) Fear of suffering—sure. Pain. Getting mauled by a bear: totally!

But more about spiritual death: *"When you give up your dream, you die,"* says Nick in *Flashdance,* my all-time favorite movie.

When you give up your dream, you die.

So, the good news is—I have never given up on my dream. And thus, I remain alive.

So, I guess I'm not dead as long as I'm working towards it.

But it goes back to the old, why is it taking so long?

HER: Well, Nancy, first of all, you know that you did not have the self-confidence or equanimity to have handled this at a younger age. You were too caught up in needing to be loved, needing so much validation through "performance." But now you are at a point in your life where you prefer to get up on stage every now and then, share a couple of songs live, and then get back down and just be, and create quietly, with yourself, and just enjoy the process (naturally, without the use of substances and the illusion of peace).

So … structure … timeline … let's get organized.

2018.

No that's too scary! Too soon!

Are you sure? Can we say the end of 2018?

What must I do by the end of 2018?

Have it recorded – ready to bring to a radio station. Know exactly what radio station you want it to be played on.

But I have no idea!

Okay, one thing at a time. You have a plan for this fall for recording. Dr. Hill told you are welcome to record a few songs in the studio at LVC since your recital audio recording somehow got muffled and didn't pan out. Anything you want to re-record. That was very nice of him. *"Vessel"* is the one song you want on the radio. That is your one song. Like the guy in the recording studio in *"Walk the Line"* said to Johnny Cash, *"… **If you had time to sing one song…one song people would remember before you're dirt, one song that would let G-d know what you felt about your time here on earth, one song that would sum you up…"*** You know the song is *"Vessel,"* Nancy.

Yes, that's do-able enough. What about "DebuDisco?" Do I want to record that one too? Or is that too much pressure and too much trying to get 7 different musicians together in fall semester and everybody's really busy with their own recitals and projects?

Maybe table "DebuDisco" till later. Don't try to do it all. It might be too much. Keep it small in terms of instrumentation for now so you can focus on just getting a solid recording. Once you meet your goal, you can go to a recording studio elsewhere and hire people to help you record all your original songs.

Okay, what about the two jazz tunes so I have something to show clubs if I want to play every now and then?

I think that's okay because it only requires piano, bass, and drums. That's easy enough to do. So, you ask Henry to play bass, Bruno to play drums, and since Ian graduated, maybe JT can play piano for you since you'll be taking jazz piano lessons from him anyway. And then see if Gabby can play flute on *Vessel* again. I think that 4 musicians (5 including you) makes more sense than trying to also do "DebuDisco" with the two trumpet players and the two back up vocalists.

Okay, so my plan is to go into the recording studio this fall, which means it will be recorded by the end of 2017. Then I can take my next steps in 2018. I will go to the Vale Music Conference to learn more and I will have pointed questions to be able to ask people.

Once I nail down a date with Dr. Hill, which I will do as soon as the semester starts, I can ask Bruno, Henry, Gabby, and JT if they would like to be part of it. And I really don't need to worry because I already learned from my recital last Spring what it's like to have people agree to play, and then not be able to, and then have to find replacement musicians. I am grateful for this experience because it strengthened me. I know how to do this now. I know how to gather other musicians, schedule rehearsals, bring everyone together and accomplish a goal.

I feel better. My first steps are planned. Hooray!

Okay, off to plan my "syllabus" for my music theory-dementia intervention. I'm excited about this too!

See you next week....

Thanks,

Nancy

SESSION POSTPONEMENT NOTE

Good morning, self. I just wanted to let you know that I need to cancel our session this morning. I'd been wondering all week how I would squeeze it in with my taking off to New Jersey this morning to visit a dear friend. Too much to try to squeeze in—need to pack up, walk dogs, stop at the store. Trust me and know that I will be here next week. Please don't judge me or tell me that I'm shirking my goals.

I won't judge you. You've come a long way, Nancy. Go see your friend who has been there for you in the darkest time of your life. Go see your friend who helped to make you a beautiful bridal shower. Go see your friend who loves to break out in song with you. Go enjoy life. I'll see you next week....

SESSION #8

....

I re-read my "session note" from 2 weeks ago and it feels so far away. I re-read the self-confidence in my voice and ask "Who is this woman talking? She doesn't sound like me—doesn't sound like how I feel today. For today I feel mildly depressed, in that "who am I to think I could accomplish such a thing" place. Self-doubt creeps in as I reflect on the past couple of weeks, the other stuff of life that has been affecting me, like James being on "night float" at the hospital and the void that I feel when he is not sleeping next to me, and the "you're a loser" tape that goes off when I realize I'm not really good at making plans with others but sometimes I don't want to make plans with others because I want to keep the space open to work on creative projects but at the same time if I keep TOO much space open then I feel lonely and disconnected and forget that I'm still a human being who needs social connection because after all, "a sense of belonging," according to the research, is the number one protective factor against suicide.

So I go to church yesterday and it feels good and then I sit with my friend, Sandi, for an hour afterwards and I am filled again with a sense of social connection so that I can now go home and walk the dogs, and make an early dinner of Chicken Parmesan for James, and then when he leaves for work at 6 pm, I am able to go upstairs to the piano room where I practice technique and in the last 8 minutes of my allotted 45 minute session, my intuition tells me to leave this 8 minutes for creativity, and I start to compose a new song. It feels good to begin to compose a new song. It's my equivalent of being pregnant. My songs are my babies. I conceive, they develop....

And they are always with me. They never have to die.

My songs are always with me, anytime. Anytime I need comfort or a laugh, I pull out the appropriate "baby."

So perhaps this is how I justify my goal. This is how I check my motive to make sure it is not about greed, or stardom or any of the non-spiritual motives that could lead to suffering.

Spiritual motive: I have children. My songs are my children. I don't want to keep my children bottled up in a room upstairs. I want them to get out in the world. I want them to go and take their own journeys, although this part is scary too, like parents are protective of their children, don't want them to get hurt, I feel the same way with my songs. When you put your songs out there, people are free to engage with them, to re-interpret them so that they may express themselves. I will have to learn to be okay with this too as this is a spiritual challenge as well. If I want to truly share my babies with the world, I have to allow my babies to go on their own path ... yes, copyright and all that stuff ... hmmm ... I'm not there yet, with this one, I must be honest. But we shall see ... I know I will have to get there. After all, didn't I go out there and interpret and play others' compositions at open mic night and Karaoke in Illinois? Didn't I borrow their babies to help me get through the pain of divorce and loss and loneliness? Shouldn't I afford others the same opportunity if they choose?

Not there yet ... but aware of this spiritual roadblock.

Okay, today is Monday. I've had my "session" so I feel better. Thank you for listening, invisible audience. I appreciate having you. And so long as you never take the place of true, human, face-to-face connection which I need for my soul, then all will be well. As long as I don't try to feed my soul by staying up on stage and never coming down to have a cup of coffee with the group, all will be well.

I'm excited for the school semester to start next week. I'm excited to be back at LVC as an alumnus who continues her education with Individual Jazz Piano Instruction! I'm excited to see all the students who were part of my freshmen cohort, and so what if I'm the same age as their parents. I'm excited to see them as they embark upon their senior year and I realize it's not just about me and my own music goals but it's also about the sense of community I have with them and I get to still be a part of that loving, music community at LVC.

Time to walk the dogs.

Thanks for listening,

Love,

Nancy

SESSION #9

....

Grace: Thank you for agreeing to have a session with me on a Friday, Dr. Pearl. I know our time is Monday, but I really needed a session today and I appreciate you accommodating me and allowing me to change things around.

Dr. Pearl: Well, I had the time available in my schedule, and if it were another client who really needed a session, and I had the time, I would do the same.

Grace: Well, thank you. Because I needed to write today. But you know I feel guilty, like I should stick to the rigid imposed, structure of once a week on Monday mornings. I also feel guilty in that I realize as I write these sessions, if it takes me a year till I reach my goal, then that will be like 52 sessions. That's a lot of therapy.

Dr. Pearl: That's a lot of therapy?

Grace: Well, I was trained in the short-term model of psychotherapy. The University Counseling Center model: 6 to 12 sessions. I was taught that most therapeutic gains are made in that time period. After that, it is diminishing returns. I was taught that in order to help clients be active in reaching their goals, it is important to set a time limit so that they will be motivated to do the work in and out of therapy.

Dr. Pearl: Hmmm ... so you believe that **"one song on the radio before I die"** *should be able to be achieved in 6 to 12 sessions...*

Grace: LOL … Okay, I see what you mean. I suppose if it was a goal that could be achieved in a short term, a goal, like "I want to be more assertive," or "I want to feel hopeful again," or "I want to increase my self-esteem," then perhaps 6 to 12 sessions would suffice. But something like "I want to have **one song on the radio before I die**" might take a little longer.

Dr. Pearl: A little longer.…

Grace: Hmmm … okay, I can accept that. But I have other things that I wanted/needed to talk about today. I made a list.

Dr. Pearl: Okay, what's on your list?

Grace: Well, number of sessions, so we've covered that, and then: the downtrodden, dementia, interpersonal isolation.

Dr. Pearl: Okay, what on your list would you like to start with?

Grace: Let's go with intrapersonal isolation. It's what's jumping out at me.

Dr. Pearl: Intrapersonal Isolation

Grace: INTRAPERSONAL ISOLATION! So, I want to expound upon Existential Theory (Yalom) here. INTRAPERSONAL ISOLATION. So, I know I've shared **FEAR OF ISOLATION**. But it's complicated. It's divided into 3 parts as you know:

1. **INTERPERSONAL ISOLATION** – feeling like you don't have the sufficient social support necessary, in your life, an important protective factor in suicidality!
2. **EXISTENTIAL ISOLATION** – the reality that in some way we are ultimately alone in that no other being can ever completely share our consciousness with us (although I would assert that spirituality and connection to the mystical can help allay this…)

   And.…

3. **INTRAPERSONAL ISOLATION** – feeling isolated from parts of ourselves

I guess that's the reigning fear right now.

I am trying to integrate my identities: psychologist/musician. Every time I set out to abandon my identity as a psychologist, something pulls me in; I have some experience that makes me see I still have a purpose, something to contribute as a psychologist so I cannot completely walk away from this identity. I guess what makes me want to walk away from it is the fear that I will never really let my identity as a musician take hold.

It took me a long time to "allow" myself to go back to school. And James said I should be proud of myself because not everyone earns a degree in music at age 52. But still, the fear that even with the degree- even though I am now a licensed, stamped, certified musician--my musician identity will always be second-rate. I fear that others will flourish in their identities as musicians while I sit back and feel like a loser who just can't take herself seriously as a musician. Who just feels like she doesn't deserve to do what makes her happy.

Dr. Pearl: So even though you are now a licensed, stamped, degreed, certified musician, you still feel like you don't deserve to be one.

Grace: No! I do! I do deserve to be one. Why not? Perhaps this is where the downtrodden theme comes in. I walk on myself. I keep myself down.

Perhaps this is why I'm so drawn to helping the downtrodden. Because I am downtrodden myself. Downtrodden of my own making. No one to blame. Just me. **FEAR OF RESPONSIBILITY** … no one to blame, not a victim, keeping myself down!!! Wow, I've just had a breakthrough.

Dr. Pearl: Sounds like you have. ☺ *You see that you keep yourself down. And in doing so, you keep yourself isolated from parts of yourself. But you have the power to change that.*

Grace: Yes, I do. Thank you, Dr. Pearl. Thanks for listening. Okay, I realize the only thing on my list I didn't talk about today yet is Dementia.

Dr. Pearl: Do you want to talk about dementia?

Grace: Not really. Not now. Let me just say that I feel a calling with dementia. That I worked on the dementia ward in the psychiatric hospital. That within psychology, this is my new passion, that there are no coincidences…when you get drawn to things, populations, there is a higher purpose. Something is calling you. I believe this. But I will say more about this later. Maybe. We'll see. I'm afraid of losing focus. But maybe it's all integrated?

Dr. Pearl: Maybe it's all integrated. Maybe when you're ready to talk about dementia, you will see how it all integrates. That seems to be your theme today … integrating all the parts of yourself. Not being isolated from yourself.

Grace: Yes. Thanks for listening.

Dr. Pearl: My pleasure. See you next week?

Grace: Yes.…

SESSION #10

....

Good morning. Well, it's a Saturday morning. Okay, so I don't have to be so rigid with regard to the day of the week for my "session." But I am still keeping sessions a week apart. I find some structure helps. Yet within the structure, I need fluidity. I find this with becoming a "real" musician as well. I had my first jazz piano lesson yesterday. And I am being structured in that I will practice a certain amount each day (20 minutes to 60 minutes; 2 hours if time allows and I am so inspired). Yet within the structure, and the focus on assignments and techniques, I allow myself fluidity, I allow the creative ideas to emerge and I experiment with them. The structured, disciplined learner must allow her artistic, creative side to flow. The artist must reign in the wild and crazy and have discipline. It's a dialectic.

So … I had left off wanting to talk about dementia. So, I will talk about dementia. Deep breath, I'm not quite ready.

Dr. Pearl: What's keeping you from being ready?

Grace: Well, I'm just having a bit of a hard time sitting still as my mind races with the to-do list of the day. Tomorrow I leave for a week with James' family sans James as he is so busy with residency. But we are going to the Outer Banks and I'm so excited because I've never been there. I'm looking forward to being in nature, and I'm looking forward to bonding time with my new extended family. But between now and tomorrow, I need to pack (which I hate … I have "packing anxiety disorder" for sure), I want to prepare some meals for James, I'd like to clean the place a little because I like coming home to a clean place, and I want to give little Charlie a bath since James says he stinks right now. Okay, breathe … I will get it all done. Whatever is important will get done. I prioritize. Right now, my session with you is what is right in front of me.

Dr. Pearl: Here we are.

Grace: Yes, just writing it down; just "speaking it" out loud removes the power of the anxiety. That is what I believe. That is my experience. Okay, 1, 2, 3. Time to talk about dementia!

So, I started "dating" dementia when I was volunteering in the nursing home. I had decided to volunteer there after I was asked to resign from a job because I had relapsed and threw up all over my office.

It was a blessing in disguise because I really didn't like that job—it was way too much pressure and it just wasn't the right fit for me. But it was a stepping stone. It was the job that got me back east, closer to home where I needed to be so as not to feel so lonely.

Anyhow, my friend was a dietician at the nursing home and suggested I volunteer there while I figure out what I was going to do next.

I became fascinated. Fascinated by the people who had conversations with me as if I were someone else. Who had conversations with people who were not visible to the human eye; they lived in a different reality than the one that us supposedly "normal" people could see. But I could connect. I could meet them where they were. I could go into their reality and be with them.

So, when I then took a job at the State Psychiatric Hospital, I shared with them this interest and they placed me on a ward of 25 men with "dementia." And when I say "dementia," I mean the term broadly, because after all, dementia was once an umbrella term to mean any kind of loss of mind—memory distortions, talking to unseen people, living in a different time/space than the physical one that is in the moment. So many possible reasons for this---physical brain damage due to accidents, drugs, alcohol, strokes; genetic variations, unresolved conflicts of the past, traumas never healed … so many differences in the varieties of possible reasons … so many similarities in the way they move through daily life.

And again, I found that I could find my way into their world and meet them and be with them.

Then, I became curious. Could I bring them back? Some of these men who had histories of being lawyers and chemists and musicians and fathers and sons and brothers. Could I bring them back?

"What's the point?" asked T.S., who spent most of his day talking to unseen people, when I was able to focus him for a moment in the here and now to do some math problems. Some of the men didn't want to be in the here and now. After all, it has been said that "unnatural dementia" is when the mind leaves the body before its time because the mind no longer *wants* to be here, but the body is not quite ready. Indeed, some of these men no longer *wanted* to be here in the material world, yet it was not yet their time to cross over.

But maybe if we give them a sense of purpose and have some fun, and help them connect while simultaneously stimulating their brains, they can come back somewhat? Maybe they would want to come back somewhat?

So, I started "Learning Community," a group of 10 men—we made it a hodgepodge high school class---a little bit of social studies, science, math ... they had fun re-learning things—they came alive. We learned and laughed together.
And then as I was embarking on my own new learning with taking an on-line music theory class, it occurred to me— "Learning Community: Music Theory." This could be my group for the next trimester. A specific course combining the fun of music and learning basic music theory to get everyone engaged. One of the interns joined me and the men really seemed to enjoy it and look forward to it.

I did some pre-testing with the group and had intended to do post testing to see if the men improved in cognitive functioning, but I left the hospital before I could do that.

So now ... now ... in my work here as a "private practitioner," I have been blessed to have a client who has survived a stroke. He has memory loss. He has difficulty with processing speed. He loves music and actually studied music many, many years ago. When I told him about my idea, he was very excited.

So, we did some pre-testing—processing speed and memory tests and now we have embarked upon a "semester" of learning music theory. We just completed Unit II. The plan is to go through the book, have him do all the lessons both in and out of session, and then we will re-test him at "the end of the semester." Will he improve? Who knows? But either way it's a win because he is enjoying it, it gives him a sense of purpose, and it helps him see that his mind can function.

So, we'll see....

The joy for me is in my identity as an applied research psychologist and as a musician. The parts of me that come together and work together. The joy for me is in watching another human being get excited about something and develop hope for his future.

I hope to take it out and do groups in other settings. That is the goal.

For now, it feels good to write about it. To let you know what I'm doing. To tell you about my sense of purpose that keeps **FEAR OF MEANINGLESSNESS** at bay. That keeps **FEAR OF INTRAPERSONAL AND INTERPERSONAL ISOLATION** at bay.

Okay, thank you for listening today. I think I'm ready to go pack (ugh!!) now.

Dr. Pearl: Enjoy packing. Put on some music. Dance around and have fun with it. ☺

Grace: ☺

SESSION #11

···

I take a deep breath and I pray. Pray to be guided. What shall I write about today in my session? What is necessary for me to "talk" about to help me reach my goal?

I'll begin with steps taken today toward the goal. (Visible, practical, measurable steps, anyway).

I talked to Dr. Hill. Hooray! Now it becomes more real and tangible because I talked with Dr. Hill about setting up a time to record my songs. He cautioned me that the piano in the studio is not that great and that I might want to have my pianist check it out and if it's not acceptable we can do the recording in one of the concert halls. I think to myself that I hope that the piano is good enough because I really like the idea of going inside to a studio where we, as Dr. Hill says, "have more control." Control.

Control. **FEAR OF RESPONSIBILITY.** What can I control? I control my effort to go in and speak with Dr. Hill. I control that I get on the computer and send emails to Henry, Gabby, and Bruno to see if they want to join me on the recording because as Dr. Hill has recommended, I should "pull my team together," and then we will figure out a time that works to do the recording.

It is the seemingly "little things" that present me with anxiety, such as sending emails. I've always been an introvert masquerading as an extrovert. So, my authentic self is shy when it comes to reaching out to others and asking them if they'd like to be involved in my recording.

Yet the anxiety is healthy. It is normal anxiety that means I'm excited about this. *If it excites you AND scares you a little, it is something you must do.* If it ONLY excites you, watch out -- you may be headed for danger. If it ONLY scares you, why bother? What are you trying to prove? And to whom?

Steps taken. Deep breath. Project set in motion.

I take another deep breath and go to a noon meditation group because I realize that I haven't been meditating as much and- as a result - I observe the craziness up in my head—the racing thoughts, constantly. Need to quiet that chatter. So, I go to the meditation group and feel the joy of connecting with others in silence. No idle chatter outside of me. And the idle chatter within settles down as well so I am free to hear the quiet voice that guides me through the rest of my day.

The quiet voice … sometimes it's G-d. Sometimes it's my mother.

I know that I am on this journey not only for me but for her as well. She is with me always. She was and is a gifted pianist who started playing the piano by ear when she was 2 years old. While I'm not much of a pianist, I am hoping that she will channel some of her spiritual energy into me when I sit in front of the piano to practice today. After all, I am here not just as me, but as her daughter, helping her to fulfill her unfulfilled dreams as well. I inherit my mother's wounds and it is my job to heal them.

I went back to school not just for me, but for her. To help her learn how to read and write music and play piano beyond just the Key of C.

And I know she is with me. She sends me signs and appears in fun ways. Like when I was walking along the beach last week and Susan is talking about her aunt who died at 57 and I share that my mom died at 54 and **at that very moment**, the back of my bikini top comes undone mysteriously, no wind, nothing to unhook it, and Susan is also amazed as my boobs almost fly out and it is as if my mother is telling me to tell them that she died of breast cancer and she is letting her presence be known by unhooking my top.

She is there. No, we can't see her with our eyes. But she is there. And I am comforted. And I laugh.

When she appears in these ways, I know there is meaning in all this sometimes seemingly meaningless life. There is **MEANING.** I am here with a purpose. Many purposes.

My purpose in this moment is to end this "session" and head to the practice room. I will pray before I play. Please, mom, channel some of your gift through me.

Thanks for listening.

Love,

Grace

SESSION #12

....

Hello self.

I'd like to begin by sharing a little more of my process with them.

Them-the imaginary audience who will one day be a real audience. For I write not just for me but for them.

So, my process is to

1) Read over the last session note, as I would with any other client, so that I can remember what I was working on, pick up where I left off, and attune to the goals, to the process....

2) Read the emails I've sent to myself. Because during the week I get an intuitive thought and I know instinctively that this is something I need to talk about with you, my therapist self. I plant the seeds, and trust that just like when I walked into the classroom with 2 or 3 goals planted in my head and trusted the process, the lesson unfolded exactly as it should. It took me a few years to come to this. In the beginning I was overwhelmed as a teacher, trying to plan and control everything. But eventually, through the process I learned that it was just a lot simpler to have the 2 or 3 goals written in front of me and then talk. It would come out ... the dialogue with students would happen naturally.

Anyhow, so I plant my seeds ... which today were reminders to myself to talk about integration and the world-as-a-psychiatric hospital. It will unfold as I write.

3) Pray. I always pray before my sessions. With others. With myself. I pray that I be guided. There is something magical and mystical about praying for guidance in everything I do. It opens up my otherwise-stubborn-vessel to hunches, ideas, and techniques....

Okay, ready, set, go.

Integration---Mary asked me what I was doing now that I've graduated music school. What was I doing as a psychologist? As a musician? I told her that I was working on integrating the two identities and that it was happening gradually. She noted that this was interesting in that after all, psychotherapy is about just that—integration.

Integration of who we are. And that connects with intrapersonal isolation---parts of ourselves we cut off and become isolated from. Although, I was never really cut off from myself as a musician. I've always been a musician. Just never felt that I had "permission" to make it my primary identity.

GRACE: Permission from whom?

ME: I was thinking about it. I could easily be a victim and blame others. I could say that I learned that music is not a safe, secure thing to do career-wise. I could blame my music teacher for encouraging me to "stick to singing" when I couldn't blow the flute and perceive through my victim lens that this was a message telling me I am not a "real" musician.

Sure, those things affect me. Yet, I know there are plenty of people who rise above messages, whether intentional or perceived, to pursue what they are passionate about. So, the permission that I've really been seeking—is the permission from myself.

Or should I say, my "superego."

If I look at things from Freud's perspective, it looks like this: Nancy: Superego—Parent figure, worried, neurotic, concerned, lots of rules.

Luna: Id – wild child, follows all impulses, no filter, out of control

Grace: Ego- works to mediate the desires of Luna and the restraints of Nancy

I choose to call myself "Grace" at times because according to some definitions, the name "Nancy" means "grace." From my perspective," Grace" is the more adult version of 'Nancy." She is more poised, even tempered, and less fearful. She can operate diplomatically and calmly.

When I call myself "Grace Pearl," I am honoring the integration of the best parts of my mother, Pearl, into my new identity of Grace. I honor my mother and imagine we are now working together as a team. So, I give her the title, Dr. Pearl, because had she grown up in a different time with a different cultural message, she could have earned this title. So, I give her an honorary doctorate and thank her for teaching me how to move beyond scared, neurotic, Nancy.

Neurotic Nancy ruled for the first 38 years of my life. Then, I'd finally had enough of my own self-oppression. And Luna was born. "What do you do with your dark side?" I asked Mario. *"You give it a name."* He told me. And he named me Luna.

So, Luna went to Karaoke and sang out her anger and her excitement. Luna flew across the dance floor that she created as she sang, and jumped across the pool table during her song and dance. Luna had no rules. She was amazing for a while. Because she helped me to release all the creativity and passion I'd kept inside. But then Luna got to be too much. Nancy ceased to exist. And Luna ended up addicted and in the psychiatric hospital.

GRACE: *There it is. Psychiatric hospital. Do you want to talk about that now?*

ME: Well, I would like to, but I sense that I am running out of time in this session.

GRACE: *Well, yes, we are almost out of time.*

ME: Yes, because Nancy is aware that there are other things on her to-do list today, like grocery shopping this morning before clients, because I want to get a chicken and a brisket so I can make a Rosh Hashanah dinner for me and James, because after all, if I am to be integrated, that includes integrating my Jewish identity.

GRACE: *Okay, so we can talk about the "world-as-a-psychiatric hospital" next time. Is there anything else you would like to say before we end our session today?*

ME: Yes. I just want to say, "thank you for listening." Because just being able to express myself, to get it all out of myself, is the thing that heals most. Just being able to talk about my integration, and share a glimpse of what happened on my way to becoming Grace, just being able to share, and have others bear witness to my experience, helps me to know that all is exactly-as-it-should-be.

GRACE: I'm glad this helps. Have fun at the grocery store.

ME: I will. And Luna will go with me too. She'll be the one singing the items on the list, and dancing her way down the aisles...

GRACE: There you go....

SESSION #13

··

Good morning, Dr. Pearl.

Dr. Pearl: Good morning, Grace.

GRACE: May I monologue for a while?

Dr. Pearl: Of course. You feel like you need my permission?

GRACE: Well, yes, because I fear being self-indulgent.

Dr. Pearl: Well, just the fact that you fear being self-indulgent probably means that you are not going to be. What would self-indulgent look like?

GRACE: Self-indulgent would be being totally self-centered with no concern about how my behaviors affect anyone else.

Dr. Pearl: So, your desire to "monologue" in this moment—is it self-indulgent?

GRACE: No.

Dr. Pearl: Well, then, monologue away...

GRACE: Okay, well, I guess I wanted to talk about the world-as-a-psychiatric hospital lens that seems to help me. I desire to be helpful and kind. And I feel that I have made progress but I realize I am human so I can still think mean thoughts—I can look at someone and judge them. I don't like when I do this. I've made progress in not acting on the thought—but I can still think it.

But when I shift my perspective, and see people as if they were patients in the psychiatric hospital, my compassion and kindness is restored. For when I worked in the psychiatric hospital, there was no judgment on my part. I saw everybody with kind eyes.

And the reality is, there really is no difference between the psychiatric hospital and the world outside the psychiatric hospital. As we used to say in the hospital, the only difference between the staff and the patients was "who had the keys." I remember one time when the CEO of the hospital was responding to a staff concern about patients using the "staff bathroom." He pointed out that it does not matter who uses which bathroom. We're all human beings. We can use the same bathroom.

We're all human beings. Human Beings Anonymous. We're all "mentally ill." On a continuum. Like everything is. Depression and anxiety are the common cold of mental illness. We all go there.

So, if I judge another, I'm judging myself. Because we are all the same. If instead, I choose to look at the world as a big psychiatric hospital, I find myself becoming kinder. I meet people where they are at, and if they are seeming particularly "crazy" or maladjusted or annoying that day, I humble myself and remember that I've been there too.

Dr. Pearl: You've been there too.

GRACE: Yes.

Dr. Pearl: You're quiet now. You're thinking. What are you thinking?

GRACE: I'm wondering if it's time to talk about my experience of being the one "without the keys?"

Dr. Pearl: Do you want to talk about it now?

GRACE: No. Not yet. I want to talk about music. I want to talk about where I'm headed.

Dr. Pearl: Tell me where you're headed....

GRACE: I am headed to **one song on the radio before I die**! And it is a fun journey! But it's more than just one song on the radio. It's about total integration of my psychologist-musician identity. I'm enjoying the challenge of learning piano. It's harder for me because I'm not so coordinated. It's really difficult for me to play one thing rhythmically in the left hand, and another thing rhythmically in the right hand. I'm kind of a spaz. But I'm practicing. Practicing 2 hours a day. And I'm proud of myself for this. Being able to focus on practicing something new for 2 hours a day. When I was getting high, I could not have done this. I could not sustain attention on anything for very long---constant flight of ideas and inability to focus.

But now, I can focus. I take breaks. 30-minute interval, then a pause to run down and kiss James or the dogs, and then back up and at it again.

I would not have James if I were still getting high. Because I'd still be a mess running around looking for someone to save me from myself.

Anyhow, I do get frustrated. But I enjoy the challenge. Working toward a goal gives me purpose. I think of all the things I want to do. I want to be a good enough piano player so that I can accompany a choir of people in assisted living situations. People with dementia. Music brings them back. It did in the psychiatric hospital. They may have been far gone in various ways, but the music, the music brings us back to ourselves.

So, I will keep practicing piano.

And tomorrow. Tomorrow I will meet JT to rehearse. To rehearse *"Vessel"* and the jazz tunes. I will pray to keep my anxiety of "it all working out" at bay and trust the process that it will all come together. Okay, I guess I'm done for now. Thanks for letting me monologue. It helps me to feel at peace.

Dr. Pearl: No worries, Grace. Enjoy the day....

GRACE: You too, Dr. Pearl!

SESSION #14

·····································

FEAR OF DEATH:

Not actual death, but metaphorical death. Fear of ceasing to exist in any given situation. Because I edit myself for fear of offending anyone (**FEAR OF ISOLATION**) but of course, if I continue to edit myself, then I actively promote my own intrapersonal isolation. I cut myself off from myself and I cease to exist. I draw further into myself and perhaps this can lead to dementia as my soul gradually withdraws and I am in my own world because I am no longer connecting authentically with those who are in the same room as I am.

Dr. Pearl: Would you like to share with our audience what you are talking about specifically?

ME: See … even that scares me. Fear of coming across as a less than perfect human being. Letting my weaknesses show. Yet, I've come so far that I know I'm supposed to share. I mean, look at me. I'm writing clearly. I make sense. I'm not all over the place and rambling and impulsive like I was when getting high.

But you see, that's part of it too. Part of what I want to share. The pot, the weed, the marijuana, the "coffee," as my friend and I in Illinois used to call it in code, wasn't all bad. At first. Before it took over and hijacked my brain. Because at first it helped me to tune out all the white noise in the brain, all the chatter, all the negative self-talk, all the fear, all the filtering mechanisms, and instead, it cleared a path for my truth and creativity to emerge freely.

I could dance around the living room and feel the energy flow creatively, without thought, I could speak my truth, I could say things that would inspire and help others. I found that just by one person (me) being high, it sparked the conversation to a level of authenticity. My being completely honest, raw, and open could facilitate this in others. It was wonderful at first.

Dr. Pearl: It was wonderful at first.

ME: Absolutely. I stopped editing myself. I was me. 100% completely authentic me. And it wasn't bad. Good came of it. I could be free from my own chains and help others to free themselves as well.

Dr. Pearl: So, if it was helping you be free, what kept you from keeping up with it?

ME: It took over. It was gradual. Slow, gradual, but it happened. Initially I would get high once or twice a week. But then it started calling me to do more and it became every night when I got home. But I guess the turning point for me was the summer I was out on the road with Lenny and I decided to take Mary Jane, who was gradually becoming my best friend, along. I was in a town I didn't know, and I realized that if I could map out where I needed to drive (to the Crosby, Stills, and Nash concert), then I could go back driving high that night. I started driving high. And then somewhere along the trip, I discovered I didn't have to wait until evening. I could get high during the day. And then eventually, I discovered, I could be high all the time if I wanted to be. And then it took over. Then getting high was no longer a choice. I was no longer in control. The substance took control of me. And that's when I started to lose my mind.

Dr. Pearl: So, you lost your mind. . . .

ME: Indeed! And to be honest with you, I never thought I would get it back. I thought I was doomed, I thought I would be "on the other side" forever. Mentally ill. Institutionalized. Dependent on society to take care of me.

But I'm not. I'm back. I'm here. And the challenge now is to share my story. But it's more than that. The challenge is to be me. To be the free me I was before it all got fucked up. To be that person who is authentic in all situations. And now I guess I'm having trouble getting there. I'm having a hard time being "real" in all situations. I find myself oppressing myself. And maybe it's not even oppressing myself. It's just that I don't know how to "jump in" when there are conversations going on. When I'm in a room of people and it's not a structured environment where everyone gets their turn to speak if they raise their hand. I don't know how to jump in.

So, for example, we were visiting James' grandmother yesterday in assisted living, and his sister, Mary, is there too, and the baby. And I find that I answer questions when asked. But I don't know how to initiate dialogue the way I used to do. I want to be the woman I was when I was a professor. Confident. Able to bring up a subject. Talk and get others to talk in a way that we all feel connected. And I just don't know how to do it. So then in my own head I become a victim. I get into this self-talk of "I don't belong, I'm just an in-law." And at the same time. I know it's not true. It's just my perception because we're all awkward and weird and his grandmother-I'm-sure-has-her-own-thoughts running-through-her-mind. I just don't know what they are. And I don't know how to reach her. I don't know how to connect. Now, if I were high, it would just happen. It would just happen.

So, I don't know, I guess I just want to get to that place where I can be the way I was *initially,* when marijuana was a catalyst, and not a demon. No, I don't mean get high again. I'm allergic to marijuana. The challenge now is to somehow inside my brain find a way to free that mechanism naturally. Whatever the hell that mechanism is. I can do it here in my writing. How do I do it with real, live people?

Dr. Pearl: Well, if you can do it when you're writing, perhaps you might want to try talking as if you are writing?

ME: Talking as if I were writing. I think that's a good idea. In fact, I just tried it. James walked in and asked what I was doing and I told him what the book was about. I told him about my fears that I wouldn't do it because I've tried to write so many times before and have given up. "Don't give up," he said.

Dr. Pearl. Don't give up.

ME: I won't give up. *"When you give up your dream, you die,"* says Nick in Flashdance. I didn't give up on finding love, and I found it. I didn't give up on pulling together a group of musicians to play a song I'd written for my recital. I didn't give up on myself when I wanted to die.

I won't give up. I will continue to walk through my fears and frustrations. Thanks for listening, self. Thanks for listening, anybody else.

Dr. Pearl: Love you.

ME: Love you, too.

SESSION #15

....

FEAR OF RESPONSIBILITY

I am responsible for:

1. Choosing people in my support team to call when I am stressed or anxious and need to process my fear.

2. Accepting that no matter how much love, guidance, or reassurance I receive from others, it is still ultimately up to me to find a way to calm myself, to soothe myself, to move through the pain of the problem and then to come up with an action plan.

3. Remembering that creative expression, such as writing, helps me to move through the pain and the frustration, as opposed to stuffing it down inside hoping it will go away, only to see it resurface unless I use creative techniques to transform the problem into enlightenment.

CREATIVE APPROACHES TO COUNSELING – that was the name of the class I developed. I trusted my intuition to guide me to a summer syllabus divided into 4 units: Writing Therapy, Art Therapy, Psychodrama, Music/Dance Therapy. As I became more and more convinced that this would work, I was able to take responsibility and design the class, propose it to my Chair, meet the Ceramics professor who kindly provided me with clay for my Art Therapy portion, create the space, create the lessons, trust the process…

Do I have such a clear vision now with **ONE SONG ON THE RADIO BEFORE I DIE?** The challenge for me is that I am not only asking for supplies or permission or classrooms. I am asking for people's time. This is harder for me.

J.T., my piano mentor, is happy to play piano for me and can do so amazingly, but he has limited time. He would prefer to come in and play his part for the recording. Dr. Hill, who is in charge of recording, says it would be better for everyone to come together at once and play at the same time, almost like recreating my recital. To be honest, I would prefer this. After all, *"Vessel"* is a song about not being alone. We are all in this boat together. So yes, bringing everyone together for the recording makes spiritual sense.

So, what if J.T. can't do it? **"Then you'll need to find another piano player,"** Dr. Hill said. And this *scares* me. More **RESPONSIBILITY.** More reaching out and communicating and connecting and trying to coordinate schedules. Yet if I want to do this, this is what I must do. I don't have a manager who can do this for me. I am *responsible.* And it scares me!!! The "what ifs" ensue ... what if I can't find someone else? What if I can't coordinate schedules? What if time keeps moving along when I'm trying to do this and all my players are no longer available because they are getting ready to graduate and busy with other things? What if Dr. Hill says, "You know this is taking too long, we offered you this opportunity, but we don't have time for it anymore?" What if 2018 rolls along and I am nowhere near having things recorded? What if I can't do this? What if I'm not meant to do this? What if G-d decides that I don't get to have **ONE SONG ON THE RADIO BEFORE I DIE** and I just have to accept this and look around at all the people who got to have a song on the radio and feel bitter and envious? Ahhhhhhh ... exhale ... exhale.

Feels good to write.

I am *responsible*.

For what I can control.

The rest ... give up to G-d, the Universe, the mystical thing that guides life....

Trust the process.

So, when I can't sleep at night like I couldn't last night, rather than stewing, I walk downstairs for some pet therapy. Lenny is sleeping so now Charlie is the one to calm me down as I pet him.

"Thanks, Charlie."

"It's okay, mom," he says. "You calm me down when I'm freaking out and shaking during the rainstorms. I'm happy to return the favor."

"Thanks, Charlie. You're very sweet."

Lenny wakes up and now both my furry kids let me pet them and provide me comfort.

I go back upstairs and plug my headphones into a binaural beats deep sleep meditation on You-tube which helps calm me down more and sink into a relaxed state. Nothing I can do about the problem right at this moment so just relax...I do and fall asleep.

I wake up. Eat my breakfast. Read my daily inspirational readings and notice that the problem has resurfaced and is gnawing at me.

So, I write. I write. I write. I wrote.
I feel better. I can trust the process of my day now, knowing that I am doing everything in my power to take responsibility for that which I control. I surrender to the unknown...

Thanks for listening.

Later,

Love you,

Grace

SESSION #16

....

FEAR OF DEATH.

Not actual death, but metaphorical death. Death of a dream, death of ambition, death of an ability to carry out the actions necessary to achieve a goal---this is my fear.

I went to music school to learn how to communicate with other musicians—to read and write music—but also how to collaborate and connect.

I've always felt like I was not entitled to be a "real musician," even though deep down I know I have been given musical gifts and while I am grateful for those, I've always felt I lack the savvy skills necessary to be taken seriously.

"You're already a professional musician. You just haven't realized it." James tells me.

Hmmm … reminds me of when I moved to Illinois, and I was so lonely, and Mike said to me "You have plenty of friends. You just haven't met them yet." And sure enough, I made friends. Two of my closest, dearest friends, a sister/daughter and sister/mother are back in Illinois. They are in my inner circle. I did indeed meet them.

So, could the same be true? Could I already be a professional musician?

Will this first piano player call me back? Will I figure out how long I should wait before calling the 2nd or 3rd one on the list that J.T. gave me because he can't do it on a weekend although he really would like to and he sounded so great playing my songs with me? Will I be able to coordinate the schedules of whatever piano player I end up with and the students who will be playing the flute, the bass, and the drums? Will they get tired of waiting and decide they don't have the time to be part of the project? Will it happen this semester or will it have to wait until spring semester and if so, will Dr. Hill tell me it's too late to do it, sorry for you luck? Do I worry too much? Do I catastrophize? Do I tend to believe that something that is so important to me could not possibly work out?

DR. PEARL: *What do you think?*

ME: I think that I worry about the things that are beyond my control—other people—when they will call back, when they will be available, their level of interest … I can control my part in things but there is so much that is not up to me.

DR. PEARL: *So what's your catastrophic fantasy?*

ME: Well, just what I said before. That somehow I would run out of time at LVC and the window of opportunity would close.

DR. PEARL: *Okay, let's just go with that. What would you do if that happened?*

ME: Well, since this is my dream. I would not give up. *When you give up your dream you die.* I would follow in the footsteps of my idol, Karen Carpenter, who along with her brother, Richard, kept persisting past setbacks in their quest to record their music. I would not give up. I would find another avenue.

I would be guided….

DR. PEARL: *You would be guided….*

ME: Of course, I would. I know I would. And even if I do something to fuck up (which I also fear), I know I would be redirected and it would still work out. G-d is like a GPS. If you don't listen and you make a wrong turn … well, recalculating … rerouting. You get there eventually. It just might take longer than you had planned.

DR. PEARL: *It might just take longer than you had planned….*

ME: Yes. And if that's the case, so the fuck what, right? I mean good things are worth waiting for. I finally had my dream wedding at age 50. I walked down the aisle to "Let it Grow" by Renaissance, something I'd dreamed of since I first starting dancing around my bedroom to that song. It happened. My fairy tale came true. I met an amazing man with whom I will celebrate my 2nd wedding anniversary next week. It happened … not when I thought it should because I fell for the myth that there is a predictable, normal, linear sequence to life, but when it was supposed to, in G-d's time.

So deep down, in my heart, deep, deep down, I believe it will work out.

Unless of course I die!

DR. PEARL: *Unless of course you die….*

ME: I which case, I will have died trying, I will not have given up, I will have tried … and you know what, as long as I do everything in my power to keep trying, and I take control of what I can … I will be okay.

DR. PEARL: *Sounds good.*

ME: Well, I better get going. We have a client in 10 minutes.

DR. PEARL: *Have a good session. Love you.*

ME: Love you, too.

SESSION #17

....

ME: Good afternoon, self. I was wondering—would it be possible to have a two-part session today? I'd like to process my feelings "before" something I'm going to attempt and then revisit with you after.

DR. PEARL: Sure. We can make time for that. Go ahead.

ME: Okay, here's the before. So after calling around piano players—Two didn't call back, one I was able to reach and he would love to do it but won't be available until after December 15th (which is when all the students have finals), it occurred to me—sure, I could wait and record all 3 songs—Vessel, and the two Jazz pieces next semester--if that is even okay with Dr. Hill—but really, deep down, what's most important to me is recording *"Vessel."* I love the way J.T. sounded playing it, and Gabby, the flutist and J.T. are both available mid-day on Tuesdays. So, I've decided I'm going to speak with Dr. Hill today and ask him if we can just do that. If he's open to it, and we can wait till next semester to record the jazz pieces, fine. But if that's too much to ask, I would be fine just recording *"Vessel."*

That's my dream. Record this one song. I will be up front with him. I won't hide. I will tell him my intention. I will be authentic.

DR. PEARL: Sounds like a plan. And it sounds like being authentic is important to you.

ME: Yes, because that is what this is all about. I will be your vessel. You can be mine. Why should I hide anything? Why should I pretend that I just want a recording of my recital for posterity when that is not my goal?

Why should I feel intimidated asserting myself to a member of the opposite sex? I wouldn't feel intimidated at all if he were a woman. But I do feel intimidated asserting myself to men sometimes. And yet, last week, I asserted myself to J.T. I was so frustrated because I was working long and hard on my piano jazz technique and I finally realized that the reason I was so frustrated was that I don't really want to be a jazz pianist. No, my goal is to be a piano player who is decent enough to write out piano parts for her own compositions and to be able to accompany a choir of clients with dementia. I found this choral selection from West Side Story and it excited me. I wanted to play it but couldn't. I showed it to J.T. and I told him what my goal was. He had me try to play it and he was able to "diagnose" that my challenge was reading the music. He recommended these books that will help with my sight reading/playing and I've been working on it this past week and I can already see a difference. I'm working toward MY goal.

(**FEAR OF RESPONSIBILITY**) I feel less pressured. It's okay that I'm at a different level. It's okay that this is still all new to me. I get to start where I'm at. James said that perhaps I was "over-performing." In other words, I compensated for my inability to read by memorizing the pieces. So, I'm learning. Just as a child learns to read---rather than reading letters—N-A-N-C-Y, I learn the process of recognizing whole words—NANCY, or in this case, recognizing whole chords instead of having to decipher each individual note. So, I'm a beginning reader at age 52 and that's okay. I keep practicing and I will be able to accompany a choir.

DR. PEARL: Keep practicing....

ME: Yes, keep practicing. I guess the same goes for communication. Keep practicing. The more I experiment with assertive, respectful, warm communication techniques, the better I get at it. And being authentic, being authentic is such a big part of it.

I want to share with you a story of what happened Monday/Tuesday. Monday I was feeling dark and depressed all day. I realized at the end of the day that the reason I'd felt depressed was that I had not authentically connected with anyone during the day. I talked to a few people here and there, but the true authentic connection was missing. So, I felt lonely. When James came home I told him about this. It felt good to just express this to him. We decided to watch a happy movie together and it lifted my spirits.

The next morning, Tuesday, I woke up and immediately felt the darkness, and the self-hatred. It was just there. Dark, lonely, I hate you, self. Then suddenly, I had a thought. I decided that my goal for the day would be to look everyone I speak with directly in the eye, to be warm and encouraging of everyone I meet, and to just connect. And I did. And I had a great day. That evening, in the meeting, I shared that while the marijuana eventually hijacked my brain, in the beginning, it actually helped in that it triggered a mechanism that allowed me to let down my guard, to be creative, to be warm and loving and to experience connection. It worked at first. I'd be lying if I said it didn't. But then it didn't. It took over, and gradually, all it did was keep me in a cycle of suicidal thoughts.

I shared that my goal was to somehow naturally manufacture in my brain that quality that allowed me to just be "me." And the cool thing is, once I said it out loud ... it started to happen.

Like last night, when James and I were out for our 2nd anniversary (Cotton) and a cardiologist that he knew named "Dr. Cotton" stopped by and said hello and I noticed the "coincidence" and pointed it out to James and I then had the courage to ask the server if she thought there was mystical significance in the fact that a "heart" doctor named Cotton stopped by on our Cotton anniversary or if it were just a mere coincidence. She enjoyed the question and shared her own belief about how she notices that every action we take impacts everything else in the universe. Authentic human connection--- me being me—she being she…and the loneliness disappears.

DR. PEARL: So, when you connect authentically, the loneliness disappears. The darkness disappears….

ME: Yes, because I know we are all connected. And when I can reach people on that level, how can I ever feel alone, or depressed, or afraid?

DR. PEARL: Afraid….

ME: Yes. Fear … underlies everything. So my plan for today is to move past fear of everything and go talk to Dr. Hill. I'm afraid but I have faith that everything will work out exactly as it should in this grand universe….

DR. PEARL: Sounds like a plan, Nan.

ME: Thank you, self. Talk to you later.

DR. PEARL: So…how did it go, Luna?

ME: You called me Luna!

DR. PEARL: Yes, I imagined you might have needed to enlist the Luna part of yourself to drum up the nerve to assert yourself.

ME: Actually, I have to confess, I did put on my high heels just in case. They helped build my confidence. Although I didn't really need the accoutrements. Just me. Just little old confident me being assertive, respectful, warm, and appreciative of Dr. Hill's willingness to allow me to record my song. So, it will happen.

So, now we have to find the right Tuesday that will work for all---Gabby and J.T. are both free between 12 and 1. Gabby and I will rehearse together beforehand; J.T. and I have already rehearsed but we can do it once more. I'll get there at 11 with the recording people to set it all up. An hour to actually record the one song should be plenty of time! Hooray! I'm really excited.

DR. PEARL: *Fantastic! You did it. You pushed past your fear.*

ME: Yes, I pushed past my fear.

DR. PEARL: *So now what?*

ME: So now what...so now I just keep writing and following the path as it unfolds. It's a beautiful day out, and it's actually tomorrow because I didn't have time to report back yesterday, so I've finished the session today. And now I am off to my piano lesson. And we'll just see what happens there ... more next session. Thanks for listening, self.

DR. PEARL: *My pleasure, Luna-Grace-Nancy*

SESSION #18

....

"Good morning, Dr. Farber. How does it feel to be on the other side?" Looks of judgment on their faces--harsh, unkind, enjoying their privileged positions of power.

I will never forget that moment. Sitting on display. Surrounded by a large circle of way too many health "professionals," taking notes, lacking warmth and concern, while I sit there feeling like Morgan Freeman's character at his parole hearing in the Shawshank Redemption. Helpless—Hopeless—It does not matter what I say. I am being judged.

"Dr. Farber, we heard you cried in group this morning!" snapped the psychiatrist critically.

Well, of course I cried, you schmuck. That is what one is supposed to do. Catharsis—let one's feelings out. Have any of you ever heard of the therapeutic factors of group therapy? Shit, I can't say anything. Keep my mouth shut. I have been demoted of my power and privilege because I've had a nervous breakdown.

I remember the kind lady down the hall, Deb, advising me, "Don't show emotion here, Nancy. Don't let them see it. They write everything down and then they will never let you out. If you need to cry, go into the bathroom and cry."

I prayed to G-d and made a promise. G-d, if you get me out of this fucked up psychiatric hospital, I promise that one day I will do my part. I will get back on the "other side," and help those

who are in this trapped position, being treated inhumanely. I
promise I will do my part.

So that's how I knew. Four years later when I received the
letter inviting me to interview at the State Psychiatric Hospital,
though initially, I didn't recognize the sign, but when the
opportunity kept presenting itself and I kept being called by
Human Resources, I realized I was being called by G-d as well.

It was time. Time to go to a place where I could be a helping
"professional," while at the same time take off the mask of
invulnerability and let others see that I was human as well.
Authenticity—No, you are not crazy, my sweet patients. We are
all crazy. Some of us are just further along the continuum at
different points in our journeys. But we are all the same.
UNIVERSALITY—the therapeutic factor of
UNIVERSALITY—thank you, Dr. Yalom for nailing those
therapeutic factors. No one walks this world alone. I will be
your vessel. You can be mine.

So, I can be the scared little girl and the confident professional
all at once. The scared little girl helps to humble the confident
professional. She keeps her ego from exploding. The confident
professional can soothe the scared little girl when she is afraid.

Like last Monday, when I was out walking the dogs, and
suddenly the darkness came over me—the dark, lonely,
feeling—boom! Out of nowhere—So the confident
professional steps in and reminds me that it's just a feeling and
that it will pass, and encourages me to think of all the other
fellow travelers who may be experiencing a moment of
darkness right now at the same exact time—and boom!

Suddenly, I'm not alone. And it's not so dark and scary. And then I start to think about how not only is the world one big psychiatric hospital, but it is HEAVEN. Right here, right now. Heaven is not some place I will go to when I leave my body. I'm here right now. My task is to learn. Learn ways to find joy, to contribute, to connect, to walk through the dark moments. In HEAVEN, I am always connected. I'm not crazy or different. I'm just part of the whole.

When my mother died, initially I felt like she was gone. That she had gone to this place called Heaven. But when she started presenting herself in mystical ways, I realized that, okay, maybe she has traveled to some cool place where she hangs out and it's her home base, but she's always flying around here and visiting and doing shit to let me know she's here. So maybe there is no place—maybe this is it and we just change forms.

I can never know for sure how it all works, but it doesn't really matter if I get it right or not.

I just have to get right what I feel is my life mission, whether this is the only life or there are more. I mean, yes, part of me believes that we just keep getting re-incarnated until we get it right and then we earn our angel wings. And there's a part of me that believes that our journeys include the mission of healing the wounds of our parents.

I have so many clients right now who are struggling to be "good" parents. So much of their identities are tied up in helping their kids be all they can be. They worry so much. My mother was the same way. She felt so helpless over my pain. It pained her when I got depressed. She worried about my social life. She wanted me to be popular and have friends. But I worried about her too. I worried that she spent so much time minimizing her talents and her brains. I worried that she cried in the bathroom and had unfulfilled dreams. That she didn't take herself seriously and dropped out of college even though she graduated high school class with high honors. I worried that she was a gifted piano player who always wanted to play in a piano bar and never did.

So, I rebelled against the advice to "not spend so much time doing your homework" and "can't you just copy one of your brother's term papers?" because it might prevent me from having a social life; I rebelled by getting a Ph.D. I did it for the both of us. Before she died, I got her blessing:

"I THINK YOU ARE GOING TO MAKE A GREAT PSYCHOLOGIST, NANCY," and "NANCY, I FUCKED YOU UP. BUT I KNOW YOU ARE GOING TO UN-FUCK YOURSELF."

Thanks, mom. Thank you for that gift.

So now it's time for me to heal my mom's wound. The gifted pianist—I went back to music school for the both of us. So now, I put aside the guitar for a while and I focus on piano. I work on moving beyond the key of C. I work slowly and steadily on learning how to read music. So eventually, my mom and I together can start a choir. And yes, mom, at some point, perhaps I will be decent enough to play at a "piano bar," here and there. Or how about we do a coffee house? Can we compromise on that? I mean, I do like that environment more and it's healthier for a recovering addict.

PEARL: WHATEVER YOU THINK, MAMALA. I TRUST YOU.

ME: Mom, you showed up!

PEARL: YES, I AM HERE. I AM GOING TO GO WITH YOU TO LVC TO PRACTICE PIANO THIS AFTERNOON. I KNOW YOU'RE HAVING A HARD TIME COORDINATING USING THE PEDALS, WHILE YOU FOCUS ON ALL THE OTHER STUFF JT IS TEACHING YOU. IF YOU REMEMBER, I WAS BIG INTO THE PEDALS AND USED THEM A LOT. I'LL HELP YOU WITH THIS.

ME: Thanks, mom. And thank you for helping me with my social skills. You were always so good at that too. I'm being more assertive and less shy and afraid. I'm being more assertive and less aggressive! I'm waiting to hear back from the student who is going to do my recording. James tells me to give him a week. Some people take longer to get back on things. So, I will be patient.

PEARL: IT WILL ALL WORK OUT, HONEY. YOU ARE BEING GUIDED.

ME: Thanks, mom. Well, it's 10:26. I said I was going to write until about 10:30 so here it is. I'm going to walk the dogs now, and then vacuum a bit. And then we'll head to LVC together.

PEARL: I LOVE YOU, NANCY.

ME: I love you, mom! ☺

SESSION #19

....

Thanks for seeing me at 5:25 AM.

HER: My pleasure—I am always here for you. I am your higher self.

ME: I know. Thank you.

HER: What's going on?

ME: Well, I woke up suddenly and realized it was an hour before I usually wake up. And I noticed that I wasn't feeling excited about the day. I was feeling afraid but I wasn't feeling excited. While I am grateful that I get to "compose" my own day, it's also challenging.

FEAR OF ISOLATION—Both interpersonal and intrapersonal.

HER: Interpersonal and intrapersonal. Which would you like to start with this morning?

ME: Intrapersonal. Interpersonal. You see, Saturday, I had this wonderful day with myself. And others. I was practicing piano at LVC. I was in the room and in the zone. And even just walking into the Music Building, I felt connected. I always feel that way there. Because others are doing the same thing as I am. I hear someone grooving on the bass guitar in a practice room, and another working on a song on the piano with vocals. And I am not alone in my aloneness because we are all in there in this magical space doing our thing.

And then I go to the library where I feel the same thing. The library has always been that wonderful safe haven for me. I mean, even when I was at the very bottom of my pit after getting out of the psychiatric hospital, and I was living in Westchester on my medical leave going to a partial hospitalization program while my friends back in Illinois took care of Lenny --I was in such a consistently dark place back then. I was so anxious and panicked all the time. I felt like I was coming out of my skin. But I remember this one day, I walked into the library there in White Plains. A beautiful, big library. I found a book and I sat at a table where others were sitting as well. I started to read, and for a few moments, I felt calm. I felt completely calm. And in that moment, I had this intuitive feeling that everything was going to be okay. That this dark pit in my life would pass. This pit was just a plot turn in my movie, an unexpected plot twist. I never expected that I would go to such a deep, dark place of suffering. But does anybody?

Anyhow, the library, that was my haven. So, Saturday, between the music and the library and doing what I loved, I felt connected. Not to mention I had plans that evening, something to look forward to with friends, out in a costume dancing my ass off with other women. Laughing, dancing, connecting—it was a perfect day and evening.

I have to be honest, just recalling the joy of the day right now in this moment, just writing about it makes me feel better already because I know there will be more days like that.

HER: *You feel better already. I am happy for you. Writing is powerful.*

ME: Yes, it is. Still, I think it's important that I talk about what I was initially thinking about at 5:25 in the morning. Because it will resurface—the "thing" always does.

HER: *Go ahead.*

ME: Well, I did wake up wondering if I would feel lonely today. You see yesterday, I didn't connect with others as much. It was Sunday, my "day off," and I was tired so I decided to keep it simple. I practiced piano because that's important to me and the only other thing I kept on my "to do" list was to open up the dehydrator that James bought me for Christmas which has been sitting there for months. I cut up apples and tomatoes because I am determined to make dried apples and sundried tomatoes. That was my project. The dehydrator seemed to be taking a lot longer than the manual said it would to dry the apples and I got frustrated. But I was also tired, so finally, after watching a couple of episodes of The Brady Bunch, I decided to go upstairs and nap for a bit before it was time to go with James to the residency dinner.

But it's hard for me to nap during the day. I get this overwhelming sense of guilt, like I should be accomplishing more, and who am I to nap, how dare I nap, I don't work hard enough to nap.

HER: Critical voice

ME: Yes, it was an inner battle. The critical voice kept attacking—you're lazy! Oh, she was relentless. But I did become aware of her so I tried to summon you, my loving higher self who doesn't judge and is patient and kind. Finally, the only way I could get through the guilt feelings was to remind myself of my personal philosophy on days that I feel useless that "If I can be of help in some way to one other human being today, then I have done my part." Then my day would have had meaning and purpose in some way (**FEAR OF MEANINGLESSNESS**). I told myself that I would be aware of this at the residency dinner and try to help the interviewees in some way.

HER: So, what happened at the residency dinner?

ME: Well, we went to pick up the candidates at the hotel, and there was that awkwardness where people are introducing themselves, and don't know what to say, and everybody's nervous and wants to make a good impression.

So, I decided to try to make things a little fun by saying, "Okay, I'm going to try to remember everyone's name" and share about a game I always use— "I'm going on a picnic" to help remember names. "I'm Nancy, and I'm bringing Noodles." And then I demonstrated that James could say, "I'm James and I'm bringing Jam." James then joked "I would probably bring Sandwiches," and I teased him back that he could not bring Sandwiches unless his name was Sam. Everyone laughed and our little Sonny and Cher routine helped make things fun, but at the same time, I found myself thinking, "No, I would really like to play the game. Not just talk about it. And if I were teaching, I would. I did. Or if I were in charge tonight, I would." But I wasn't in charge. It wasn't MY residency dinner. I am just the spouse. I don't have a professional identity here this evening. I am a spouse.

And this gnawed at me throughout the dinner. While I do think I was successful in helping lighten the mood, and I was just Nancy, being funny, and helping others to laugh during what can be a nerve-wracking experience—I was very aware that no one knew I was a psychologist, or a professor, or a musician. They knew that I was James' wife. And then as James and his colleagues talked about the day-to-day of the medical center, and their team, and what a great group they have, and all the exciting things they are learning, I found myself feeling envious.

HER: Envious.

ME: And fearful.

HER: And fearful.

ME: Fearful that perhaps I'd made a bad decision by going on this unknown path of "composing a life." Where I don't have a place to go every day where I see the same people and have a sense of belonging. Fearful that maybe I'm not strong enough to be living this new chapter of my life in which connection and purpose is not ready-made for me at a structured place where I show up. There are no automatic connections that are consistent on an everyday basis. I have to work to create them. Fearful that because there is not "one place" where I show up and I am known, like as the professor at the university, or the psychologist at the hospital, that I will somehow lose my professional identity because there are no people consistently mirroring back to me who I am.

Hmmm....

HER: *What are you thinking now?*

ME: I'm channeling Nick from Flashdance again. "When you give up your dream, you die."

HER: *When you give up your dream, you die.*

ME: **Follow your dream, Dr. Farber!"** I remember the words of one of the patients as I announced that I was leaving my job and going back to music school. Follow your dream. So, I guess, I'm realizing that even though there are moments where I feel lonely and I doubt myself, I have to keep following my dream. I could go back—there is always a Plan B. if I had to go back, I would. For now, though, I believe I am to work through the challenge of creating community.

I am a professor. I am a psychologist. I am a musician. I am a wife. I am a dog mother. I am all these things. I do not have to lose parts of myself. I carry them with me.

So, in this challenge of creating community, creating my "workplace," I am aware that I have lunch plans with a colleague today who is going to give me some feedback on the senior living places she visited for her parents. She thought of me when she visited them and mentioned my music plans. She noted that they were interested in the idea. So, you see, I am connected. My workplace is just a little more spread out and requires some tools for navigating. My workplace is my office, LVC, the library---my workplace is Subway where I will meet my friend for lunch today.

HER: Your workplace is everywhere you go.

ME: Yes...

HER: Yes....

ME: I'm tired. I feel better. Thank you for listening. I think I'll go back to bed for a little bit.

HER: Sounds like a plan. ☺

SESSION #20

ME: Good afternoon, Dr. Pearl. How are you today?

DR. PEARL: I am well. Thank you for asking. You seem like you are in a good mood. What's going on?

ME: I am in a good mood. I'm in the library right now. It feels good to be writing in the library. After all, if one is writing a book, is not the library a logical environment to write in? My workplace is broadening. I have been feeling more connected … and more integrated.

DR. PEARL: More connected … more integrated.

ME: Yes, and I feel like the balance of psychologist/musician/wife is coming together more.

Oh, I have to tell you. I have a date for the recording. December 5th---we will record *"Vessel"* on December 5, on a Tuesday. And James was right…I had to be patient. People get back to you. Be patient. That is a hard one for me. Actually, I'm embarrassed to admit that I did let my impatience and fear get the best of me yesterday.

DR. PEARL: What happened?

ME: Well, you see, I had to get my computer fixed a couple of weeks ago, and I was actually somewhat patient with that process—I borrowed James' old computer while mine was in the shop.

I was grateful that I had a substitute computer to use while I awaited the long process of the computer folks diagnosing, re-diagnosing, and then finally being able to target and repair the problem that was making this white fuzzy, screen come across my laptop. I had even told myself, "Nancy, don't worry, worst case scenario, you buy a new computer. *It's only money*; just accept whatever is."

But when I got my computer back, and I was doing my monthly Medicare billing on Friday, I noticed that after the computer folks reloaded all the software, I couldn't get the CMS 1500 form to line up--the printout was all misaligned. I emailed Dan, the man from whom who I purchased the 1500 template, because he had helped me with this very same problem when I initially set it up. I asked if I could speak with him that afternoon. Dan emailed me back and suggested I print out a "John Doe" form he had sent, see how it prints, and then scan it and email it back to him. He would then adjust it for me.

But of course, I went into panic mode. I was worried about it because I like to do my billing at the end of the month, and now I would be behind. James suggested that I just let it go, enjoy the weekend, and deal with it on Monday. It was already after 5:00 on Friday.

Well, that was good advice. I calmed down and I did enjoy the weekend. But then Sunday early evening, as we were getting ready to go to another residency dinner, for some reason, I thought, "I need to deal with this now."

Fear came over me. Fear of "what if I never get this fixed and cannot bill for Medicare sessions," which of course leads to fear of running out of money, and then I'm in the homeless shelter and ultimately of course it connects to **FEAR OF DEATH**.

Although when I was "on the other side," my therapist, Susan, said to me "Nancy, if you were in a homeless shelter, you'd probably start a choir there." Perhaps.

I guess though, that I was mostly worried about not having enough time to do the other things I wanted to do on Monday, like working on a proposal or just organizing my ideas before I call one of the assisted living places to talk about my music groups. There were things I really wanted to work on and I was afraid I would not have enough time.

DR. PEARL: Afraid you would not have enough time.

ME: Yes, Good old fear. Because of course if I run out of time, or rather, if things don't happen in the timeline that I expect them to, then my life is meaningless, because my life's purpose is now wrapped up in just figuring out how to print out forms from the computer.

I know. I laugh as I realize how ridiculous this is.

DR. PEARL: It's okay, Nancy. We need to learn the same lesson over and over until it really kicks in. Patience is a life lesson for you. You fear running out of time and not accomplishing your goals. You **fear** *MEANINGLESSNESS.*

ME: Yes, but anyway, what I wanted to share was that I decided to try to scan the document right then. But then I couldn't even get the scanner to work. I got so frustrated with nothing working that I started to take it out on James.

"Why are you yelling at me?" he asked. And of course, I said, "I'm not yelling AT you. I'm just yelling because I'm frustrated. You just happen to be here in the room."

But still, the yelling affected him. It made him uncomfortable. That's not fair to him. And while I wasn't yelling "at" him, I kind of was, because I was begging him to help me figure out how to fix the problem. And as he noted, he's not tech savvy, but still he was trying his best to help me, and to calm me down.

Well, we were finally able to get the scanner to work. So, with a piece of the problem resolved, I was able to calm down and go to dinner.

The next day, I emailed Dan back with the scan. He emailed me back with instructions on what to do next. Again, it wasn't working at first, but I stayed calm until I figured it out. And Voila! My Medicare form printed out perfectly and my life is back on track.

DR. PEARL: *So, your life is back on track. So, what is the point of the story? Tell them.*

ME: The point of the story is that inner peace leads to world peace. I mean think about it. I get frustrated. Frustrated---I am not aware in the moment that underlying this frustration is fear. My fear turns into frustration turns into anger. I take this anger out on someone else.

Fortunately, the damage could have been worse. I am able to say "I'm sorry" and make amends to James.

But the damage could have been worse. Multiply my frustration and lack of self-awareness. Multiply my fears. What do we see then?

> Bullying
> Bombings
> Mass shootings

Inner Peace leads to World Peace

Not my idea; heard this from Lauren, the woman who helped me when I was going through my divorce.

Then, again, there really is no such thing as a completely original idea, is there? We each have the ability to discover ideas in our own way. We can each express ideas in our own creative way.

So instead of competing over who "had the idea first," and who "stole my idea," perhaps it's better to just accept that we are all connected, we all have the same fears, and we can all make our own unique contribution to this world in how we creatively express ourselves.

But we must heal our fears. We must notice them. So that they don't turn into anger, into hate, into suicide, into homicide.

DR. PEARL: Suicide; Homicide.

ME: Yes, if we do not heal the fear, if we do not heal the hate within us, we take it out on ourselves or we take out it on others. And sometimes we do both. So, I guess I just want to play my part in the healing. We all have a part to play. .

DR: PEARL: Yes, we do.

ME: Well, thanks for listening. I am going to work on being more patient. More gentle. I wash all my clothes on Gentle Cycle. I want to apply this to everything.

DR: PEARL: Gentle. Well, have a gentle rest of the day, Nancy.

ME: Thank you. See you soon.... ☺

SESSION #21

....

Many paths can lead to the same destiny. While I tend to worry sometimes about what I'm doing—Am I on the right path? —I do have this intuitive hunch that all paths will lead me to the same destiny. That even if I seemingly "fuck it up," or make what I perceive to be a "wrong turn," or a diversion, I still get to the same place, the place I am headed in my life.

It's like religion or theoretical orientation. I mean there are so many religions out there—and yet, they are all really trying to do the same thing: provide us with comfort, with a road map for being a good human being and for tapping into the mystical power beyond us that intervenes in our lives in magical ways and guides us; help us to accept what is beyond our control; help us to find meaning in life; teach us how to love. It doesn't matter which one you pick or if you come up with your own belief system, no matter which path you take, you will get there ... (where?) Ha, ha, ha ... You can decide that too. To where is it you are ultimately trying to get? Is it to a place? To a goal? To a feeling of serenity?

I feel the same way about "theoretical orientation" when it comes to practicing as a psychologist/therapist. It doesn't matter what your theoretical orientation is---you will get there in helping your clients meet their goals—many paths to the same outcomes, whatever that desired outcome may be.

So, my personal "theoretical orientation," has always been primarily "existential." When I first read about "existential theory," it just clicked with me. When I read about the 4 givens of existence-**death, responsibility, isolation, meaninglessness**- I knew in my heart that this was what I believed about the fears that underlie the human condition. Yet I am "technically eclectic" as they say. And I am aware that there is more than one way of conceptualizing the challenges to the human condition and suffering. We just have to find the lens that fits for us. For me, existential theory poses the questions, the problems to be addressed. For me, many of the answers come from spirituality....

And creativity.

"If I don't create, I will die." Those were the words of my friend Bryce, the pastor/artist who was also a regular at Jackson Avenue Coffee, my home in Charleston, Illinois.

Jackson Avenue Coffee was where I would sit and write, where I would sit and read my students' papers and accidentally spill coffee on them so that I would then have to apologize for the coffee stains as I returned their papers. Jackson Avenue Coffee was the place where on Thursday nights, I got to experiment at Open Mic Nite. With my guitar. And my songs.

"What are you performing tonight, Nancy?" the kids would ask. "No, it's not a performance," I would say. "It's an expression." I'm not performing because for me, the word "perform" places some kind of inauthentic pressure on me, that I am here to entertain in a way with the intention of accomplishing a certain outcome. No. I am expressing myself.

Expressing myself creatively.

I would try out my original songs at Open Mic Nite. Others would do the same. It was our safe haven to experiment and express ourselves.

I miss the JAC. I love the JAC. But everything changes. And we must find our new homes.

So now I live in Pennsylvania and I decided last week to experiment with my newly developing piano identity and my interpretation of "And Your Bird Can Sing" by the Beatles. I expressed myself at Open Mic Nite in Annville. A bunch of the LVC students were there and the girls cheered me on which felt good. *I am connected.* I am accepted.

I was happy. But I realized that something was different within me. Now that I am a certified, stamped, degreed "musician," I worry more about how my self-expression is being received or evaluated. Yes, I guess "performance pressure" kicks in. I hold myself to a standard that I've created in my mind and I imagine that others are doing so as well. They may be. They may not be. I have no idea what's going on in their minds. Does it matter?

At one point, I messed up the piano part and just restarted the phrase again. Then I kept going with even more expression and feeling than I had before the mess up and I felt good. But...what did others think? How would I know? After talking with my friend, Trish, fellow psychologist and graduate school classmate, she reminded me of a reading in a book we used for a class we taught—Hamachek's *Encounter with Others*—"We like those who are competent yet who blunder."

Competent and they blunder. Makes sense. We want to admire people yet we want to see that they are human too. Nobody can be "perfect" all the time.

So now I've decided that it's time to bring Pearl (my guitar, named after my dead mother) to Open Mic in Annville. I want to play "Vessel." I want to play "Sunbird." I want to play my creations. I want to express myself and have others bear witness to my self-expression.

I'm listening to the Beatles right now as I write. They inspire me. Musicians inspire other musicians. When we are creative, we inspire creativity in others.

So, this past weekend in Cleveland, I was inspired. By a pair of musicians at The House of Blues. And a woman creatively expressing herself in the bathroom. And Dirty Dancing. And a song on the radio in the Ubermobile.

James and I were riding in the Uber on the way to meet his colleagues for drinks and appetizers before hosting their booth at the Family Medicine conference. The song "Sister Christian" was playing on the radio. "Be a Sister Christian," I thought to myself. Be kind and loving and don't worry so much about feeling like an appendage when you are with James and his colleagues. You will find your way to connect. To matter. To exist.

And sure enough, I did. There was another woman who was also somewhat of an outsider because she worked at a different medical practice in another part of the state. She was grateful that the group had included her in their gathering. And I chatted with her. And as I allowed myself to connect, James pointed out to me that the song Sister Christian was playing again--on the radio in the restaurant! Mystical coincidence assuring me I am on the right path. Be a Sister Christian, Nancy. Show loving kindness to another human being.

After drinks and appetizers, we all squished into an Uber together. It was really, really, cold outside and it seemed that we were all enjoying being squished into warmth and I found myself connecting with James' colleague on the topic of Irish Coffee and how it warms you on so many levels.

I got triggered. I found myself craving an Irish Coffee. But I was able to play the tape through and imagine where the Irish Coffee would take me—to another Irish Coffee, and then only a matter of days until I'm justifying finding marijuana somewhere, and then maybe getting high again a month later, and then a week later, and then a day later, and then an hour later, and then my life is a big smoky haze and I lose motivation and I can't function without getting high and all my goals and dreams are lost.

So, instead, I decided to find a hot chocolate. I announced my plan to find a hot chocolate to my Ubermates and bid them goodbye as they headed for their booth at the conference and I headed for some time with myself. As I walked back to the hotel where James and I were staying, I couldn't find a coffee shop but then thought "maybe they will have a hot chocolate in the hotel restaurant."

Indeed. I ended up sitting at the hotel bar, drinking a hot chocolate out of the same type of glass they serve Irish Coffee in. My pseudo-Irish Coffee complete with whipped cream and a cherry on top. And as I sat drinking my beautifully decorated hot chocolate, talking to the bartender about her big win in the casino, feeling so grateful that I no longer needed to depend on a mind-altering substance to connect, I knew again that I was being guided. And that I was on the right path.

After my hot chocolate, I decided to go up to the hotel room and just relax for a bit and watch some television. One of the nice things about not having cable television is that when I go to a hotel, I thoroughly enjoy all the television choices. It is such a treat!

So, I lay down in my comfy hotel bed for a while, tuning into the last half hour of "Nobody puts baby in a corner" and smiled ear-to-ear as Baby did the lift and her dad beamed with joy and said "When I'm wrong, I say I'm wrong" to Johnny. Fully fulfilled and inspired, I was ready to go out. James would be done at 9:00. It was 8:30. I'll get a head start. I could walk around downtown and head into the House of Blues where James and I had planned to go. It's okay if I get there first by myself. I used to go out by myself all the time.

And I did. And I felt like my old self. Sitting there, drinking a coffee, talking to the busboy about Hershey, PA, and how his dad goes there on business but he, himself has never been, enjoying the music, enjoying the realization that James would be joining me and I'm so grateful that G-d has sent me such a wonderful man and the realization that I can also be with myself and the music and that I can be in a relationship without losing myself. And I sent James a text: "At the House of Blues. Come over when you're done." And I felt great! Old, confident me....

But then of course, it was 9:00, and then it was 9:15, and then it was 9:20, and James was supposed to be done at 9:00. So, all the crazy tapes start playing in my head. No, no, no. Calm your ass down, Nancy. And I gave myself until 9:45. If you don't hear from him by 9:45, you can make your next freak-out-inspired move.   And once I gave myself a time, that seemed to help because sure enough, at about 9:30, he texted back that he just saw my text and was excited to come meet me at the House of Blues.

So ... after James showed up---and now I'm really happy, because I have my James, my music, and my me, and I've diverted a freak out-- something really cool happened.

I had to pee so I went to the bathroom and I'm in the stall and I hear a young woman outside saying something and I thought she might be talking to me but wasn't sure and I go out to wash my hands and she looks at me and says, "Hey you didn't answer my question!" So, I ask her what her question was. "Hashtag-relationship goal!" she emotes. "#Relationship goal! What is your relationship goal?"

And I find this interesting as I'd just been thinking about this and I share with her, "Well, I'm in a beautiful relationship with my husband. And my relationship goal is to keep this beautiful relationship without losing myself."

At that moment, she smiles and jumps with joy and shouts, "You are everything!" She gives me a big hug and shares with me that she's a very independent person and she's struggling with how to still be independent and be with her wonderful boyfriend. She shares with me that she is having an amazing evening with her boyfriend at the concert going on upstairs and that they actually met at a concert of this same band. I tell her I am with my man in the bar watching an awesome guitar and vocal duo and also having a great night. We laugh and share a moment. I go back outside to James and tell him of my cool experience connecting with this woman at a point in time when we were both thinking about the very same thing. It's so surreal that it doesn't feel real. I wonder if she is an angel or an apparition.

James and I sit and I enjoy the music. I order a slice of Key Lime pie and we enjoy that together as well. Then about an hour or so later, I have to pee again so I go back to the bathroom. As I come out of the stall, there she is again! My new angel/apparition friend. Either this is a mystical coincidence or we are both just on the same pee schedule. I choose to believe the former.

I write down notes on a napkin. Notes of things I want to remember about the evening. Because it is just one of those evenings. One of those evenings where I know I'm being guided. Where I know something bigger than myself is guiding all of this. So how can I ever doubt my path?

Twists and turns and signs and angels along my everchanging path. Our paths intertwine.

I am connected.

We are all connected.

Connection replaces addiction.

FEAR OF ISOLATION. At bay. **FEAR OF MEANINGLESSNESS**. At bay.

Thanks for listening.

Later,

Love,

Nancy ☺

SESSION #22

....

When you're given a second chance at life, you want to make the most of it.

"You were saved for a reason. You better do something about it."

That's what the police officer said to me. The police officer who gave me a ride from the hospital to the police station in Marshall, Illinois where I was fingerprinted, asked to pee in a cup, mug-shotted, humiliated, humbled.

"You were saved for a reason. You better do something about it."

My amnesia lifted in the hospital in the late afternoon. I'd been hit by a semi about 6 am.

"I need to talk to you about something we found in your car," the police officer said.

DR. PEARL: You paused. What's happening right now?

ME: I'm wondering how much of the story to tell? Do I tell it all?

DR. PEARL: You know the answer to that. Be vulnerable. Be real.
There's nothing you've experienced that another human being has not.
There's no thought you've had that another human being has not.

ME: True.

Well, he talked to me about the marijuana and the pipe he'd found in my glove compartment. He was looking for my insurance card after getting a hold of my brother, Matt, my emergency contact. The officer found the insurance card. And the weed. And the "paraphernalia."

The irony was that I wasn't high when I was driving. Not that I hadn't been before. But it was still in my system. I had smoked the night before.

The irony was that I was clear and alert as I drove slowly and carefully in the blizzard at 5 am on the interstate, determined to make it to the Indianapolis airport and fly to Florida for my friend's wedding. Of course, I was planning to get high in the airport before my flight took off. I was past the point of worrying about the risk of getting caught. I was invincible. I was addicted.

Then BOOM!

Suddenly I'm in a dreamlike state---smiling and feeling like I'm in a slow-motion spin.

The next thing I remember, I'm in an ambulance lying down and asking for my dog, Lenny. I cannot calm down until one of the paramedics calls the kennel where Lenny is staying and assures me that Lenny is okay. I slip back into being awake yet unconscious.

Then suddenly I'm in a hospital room—confused. Thinking I'm still married to Mike. Begging loudly for a social worker to talk with because I'm aware that I'm experiencing temporary amnesia and need someone to help me. There is no one on duty I'm told. It is a Saturday. No mental health professionals available. I am told to calm down. I am disturbing the other patients.

DR. PEARL: Go on.

ME: Well, I can't remember how and when I learned of all the details of the accident. But the story is that I was driving on the interstate in the blizzard, my car hit black ice and slid into the lane next to me. A semi-truck was driving along and tried to avoid hitting me but could not.

The semi hit my car on the driver's side. My car spun out of control. A witness, my angel, who happened to be on the highway at the time, and happened to be a paramedic, pulled me out of my car and saved me.

After the police officer came to the hospital and handed me my four tickets, he was kind enough to take me to where my car had been towed. I got to see my snow-covered smashed car... I was stunned.

It was impossible. How could I be alive? The passenger side was completely smashed in. How could I be alive? What other angels were present that morning? My mother, I'm sure. My mother. I'm sure.

"You were saved for a reason. What are you going to do about it?"

DR. PEARL: Okay, Nancy. What are you going to do about it?

ME: Well, I'm going to finish this book. I'm going to play
"Vessel" (and "Sunbird") at Open Mic in Annville tomorrow.
I'm going to practice the hell out of piano today and keep
persevering despite my self-proclaimed "piano skills disability"
and piano-special-education-student classification. I mean we're
all "special education" students in some way. We're all disabled
in some way. If we weren't, how could we ever experience
humility. "He who is exalted shall be humbled." "He who is
humbled shall be exalted."
*DR. PEARL: So, where do you need to be humbled? And where do you
need to be exalted?*

ME: Humbling. Hmmm...where has ego been my downfall?
Many places. The need to be "the best." I am not "the best." I
am only the best at being me. But there will always be more
skilled writers, teachers, musicians. I open myself more to learn
from others. EVERYONE has something to teach. Just tune
in. And when they annoy me in some way, tune in even more
closely. There is something to be learned.

I have not been successful in collaborating with others in the
past. My ego always got in the way. It had to be my idea, my
way.

But now, I strive to be more open. Like last week, for example,
I was rehearsing with Gabby. She was playing the flute part I
wrote for *"Vessel."* She asked if she could make a couple of
changes in it. Too many notes going too fast. Sounded a little
"hectic."

Of course, Gabby. You're the flutist. I don't know anything
about playing a flute. I just wrote something that fit
harmonically. So, Gabby makes some changes. We work at it
back and forth. I am not controlling. I welcome her input. And
it comes together. She thanks me. I thank her. And you know
what? There is more joy in that than in having it be "my way."

DR. PEARL: Joy in collaboration.

ME: Yes. And I never thought I'd get there, to be honest with you. I was always very protective of my own ideas and did not work well with others. I didn't want to do group projects for fear of having my ideas watered down. But where does this leave me? Lonely and disconnected. ISOLATED. The great and powerful Oz.

Perhaps I needed to be humbled. To be brought to the point of desperation where I so needed other human beings to help me. To be on "the other side."

DR. PEARL: Okay, Nancy. So, you continue to identify and work on where you need to be humbled. Good job. So...where do you need to be exalted?

ME: Hold on. Let me get some coffee and think about that.

DR. PEARL: Okay. I'll wait.

ME: I probably should stop writing. I need to walk Lenny and Charlie.

DR. PEARL: No. No. No need to avoid. Just get some coffee and take a break. I'll wait.

ME: Okay.

. . . .

ME: I'm back.

DR. PEARL: Got your coffee?

ME: Yes, it tastes good. I'm so grateful that I drink actual coffee now! Not "coffee" as in the nickname that we used to masquerade marijuana!

Although, I do need to cut back on my caffeine. I am drinking more decaf. And tea. Want to be healthy. Want to live long and well so I can write more.

DR. PEARL: Write more?

ME: Yes, I thought about it. And I must say it out loud. I am a composer. Not just of music but of words.

In fact, JT is an awesome teacher in helping me discover that when I make up lyrics to a piano tune in my special education piano book, it helps me to play better. I am a lyricist. And this book, these words that I write here, they are lyrics. My life is a sing-a-long. It is a musical comedy drama. I write the tune and the lyrics.

So where do I need to be exalted? In saying out loud "I am writing a book that I will share with the world" (or more humbly, with whomever wants to read it, if you don't like it or want to read it, that's okay too!)

You see I've written so many "books" that I've never shared. And I have not had the self-confidence to share them. So when I drove across the country with myself at age 28, and talked into a tape recorder, and transcribed everything, and combined that with my notes in my journal, and went through a process of self-discovery that I wanted to share…and then went to a writing group for novelists in The Village…and this one woman in my group really liked my book until she found out it was a true story because she really "wanted it to be a novel," and so I.…

Shelved it. As I have my other writing projects.

But perhaps they are not really shelved. Perhaps they are all practice. Like practicing the piano. Perhaps the book I am writing now is the one I am to share and the others are all "rehearsals."

I choose to believe that.

So there. I've said it out loud. This is where I long to be exalted. To be offered the confidence to say: "This is my book. I share it with whomever would like to read it."

And I will.

DR. PEARL: And you will.

ME: And I will.

DR. PEARL: And I will. We all have a "book" in us. This is mine.

ME: This is ours.

SESSION #23

....

The Four Givens of Existence:

FEAR OF MEANINGLESSNESS
FEAR OF ISOLATION
FEAR OF DEATH
FEAR OF RESPONSIBILITY

It is this last one that I believe I tend to talk about the least. And yet it is so important. For it underlies all behavioral change. Any goal I strive to reach requires that I take responsibility for my own actions. No one can do it for me. I am responsible.

So if I want to be healthy, I have to make healthy choices—in what I eat, in my "sleep hygiene" habits—like forcing myself to put the iPhone on the other side of the room, away from the bed, because I've noticed the correlation between keeping my face in the phone and racing thoughts. Reading...a book...the old-fashioned way ... quiets my mind.

I make the choice to push my comfort zones to make a phone call to set up a meeting that puts me on the path toward reaching a goal:

I am excited because I have my first "informational meeting" set up with a man from an assisted living facility this week. I'm going to gather some information about how they do things there. And I will tell him about my two groups that I want to do in an assisted living facility—Music Theory for Cognitive Stimulation and The Choir for People with Dementia.

Of course, I'll have to come up with some fun name for the choir when I do it. That will depend on the residents. Perhaps they will help me come up with a name. But I do know that it will help them. Because I've seen it help at the Psychiatric Hospital. That not just singing, but having a goal to work toward, working towards "putting on a show" helps to inspire people, helps us come alive. We must have goals. Thank you, Mrs. Banovic, my 9th grade Spanish teacher, who went on to become Dr. Banovic, for modeling this and for saying to me, "Nancy, you must always have goals...."

I am responsible. I am responsible. I am responsible.

I am even responsible for my own validation.

I discovered this last week at Open Mic nite. Yes, let me tell you what happened.

So, I went to Open Mic as planned with my intention of playing *"Sunbird"* and *"Vessel."* I almost didn't go. I almost made an excuse—too tired, too late, too nervous ... yada, yada, yada. But no. I was ready. And I was already in Annville having gone to Gabby's flute recital which was fantastic. No, I'm going to do this.

I'm going to persevere even though I feel a little awkward because it's not Jackson Avenue Coffee in Illinois, and I'm not a "regular" there and I feel different now that I'm supposedly a "real musician." No. I have a goal. I want to get back out there with my songs. Something intuitively has been telling me to do this. Follow your intuition....

So, I got up there. I really wanted to sit on the floor because I am much more comfortable sitting on the floor cross-legged when I play the guitar. I feel more connected to the guitar that way. We are one.

But the set-up wasn't conducive to that so I went with a chair which I have done before.

I started playing *"Sunbird."* And the guitar felt far away. But I managed. My playing wasn't the best. As I finger-picked I noticed that I could hear the bass string but it was hard to hear the other strings ringing out. Still I persevered. I felt good about my vocals. It wasn't horrible. It wasn't awesome. It was what it was ... at least in my perception. I have no idea what others were perceiving. Did it matter? I felt good that I played *"Sunbird."* Hadn't played it in public in years. Not since Illinois.

When I finished *Sunbird*, there was silence. Of course, I was expecting applause. But most people weren't even paying that much attention. They were on their cell phones and computers. They may not have noticed the song was over.

So, I just kind of giggled, said "That's it!" and went on to play *"Vessel."*

I could have chosen to be crushed. I could have chosen to say, "Oh my G-d, nobody clapped. How awful. How terrible!"

Nah ... I decided to validate myself instead. "Good job, Nancy. You did it! You played *"Sunbird"* after all these years. You made it through the whole song! Proud of you."

I validated myself. I am responsible for my own validation. Anyhow, I did go on to play *"Vessel"* and felt very connected with that one. I felt good.

Interestingly, later, after this guy, who wasn't a student, played Chopin on the piano, and I told him how great it sounded, he said to me "I really liked your music too. Do you write your own stuff?"

Hmmm ... so maybe some people did pay attention ... maybe some didn't ... maybe some liked it ... maybe some didn't ... we never really know how we are being perceived.

Does it matter? Perhaps a little. I mean we all seek approval externally. We crave that external validation. And perhaps if we had absolutely no external validation, something would be amiss. And then we might need to look at what we're doing.

But I am responsible for my own validation. And I am responsible for working on the things I want to improve. I could certainly practice guitar and get better at finger-picking so that it holds up under pressure. Right now, I'm focusing on practicing piano. And it feels good. Working towards a goal. Anyhow, goals. So, a week from today we will record "*Vessel.*" I am responsible for the part I am responsible for. The rest is up to the Universe....

Thanks for listening.

Later, Love,

Nancy ☻

SESSION #24

....

Miracles happen. Miracles do happen.

My furry baby boy, Lenny, turned 14 last week.

For the past couple of years, Lenny has had a harder time with long walks. We've been getting up to a mile each morning, but by 1.2 miles, he's pretty much done and ready to go back inside.

But the morning of his 14th birthday, something magical happened in Lenny. As I rounded the corner back to our door at 1.2 miles, he pulled. **"No, mommy, I'm not done. I want to keep walking."** Okay, Lenny. Charlie was done so we dropped him off and Lenny and I kept walking. We got up to 2 miles. Back to the door. **"No, mommy, I'm not done."**

Really, Lenny?!

Lenny and I ended up walking 2.5 miles that morning. And then later that day he decided he wanted to walk another mile. So, Lenny walked 3.5 miles on his 14th birthday. His birthday re-birth! And then this morning, even though for the past year Lenny has tried and tried and has just not been able to jump up onto the couch where he likes to hang out, James awoke to discover Lenny nestled up on the couch. Hooray, Lenny!

Miracles do happen.

Miracles do happen.

Nine years ago, a 43-year-old woman wanted to kill herself because she could see no way out of the darkness and the pain. Today, she awakes each morning excited about what the day will bring and is currently nestled on the couch between her two dogs as she writes.

Miracles do happen....

I'm scared and excited about the recording of *"Vessel"* on Tuesday. Scared and excited. That's always a good thing. Remember, if it just excites you---be careful ... something you're not paying attention to that you should. If it just scares you—don't bother. You don't have to prove anything. But the things that scare and excite us. These are our callings. At least that's been my experience....

The scared part. The "What ifs." What if, what if, what if.... What if someone can't make it? What if my voice or a guitar string cracks? What if it sounds discombobulated? What if the levels are off and there's no way to adjust it? What if? What if? What if?

DR. PEARL: I think it's time we did a little Gestalt exercise with the what ifs....

ME: I think you're right, Dr. Self.

DR. PEARL: Okay, who do you want to start with—the "What If's or you?

ME: Hmmm ... I'm not sure. Hmmm ...... Let's start with me.

DR. PEARL: Okay, so for the sake of doing a real Gestalt two -chair exercise, I'm going to have you move seats as you do this. Where would you like "Me" to sit?

ME: Over there, in the rocking chair.

DR: PEARL: And the "What Ifs?"

ME: Let's have them sit at the table.

DR PEARL: Okay, I'd like you to move over to the rocking chair, and begin talking/writing as yourself.

ME: Okay…Can I get some coffee first? I need a break.

DR: PEARL: Get some coffee.

……………………..

ME: Okay, I'm here in the rocking chair. With my coffee. Decaf. I've had enough caffeine for the morning.

DR PEARL: Smart choice. Okay, are you ready?

ME: I think so.

DR. PEARL: Okay, I want you to begin by just talking "to" the "What If's." Look at them over at the table. Tell them what you're feeling. Talk TO them. Ready?

ME Yes.

DR. PEARL: Begin….

ME: Hello, "What Ifs." How are you today? So anyhow, I'm looking over at you guys. You look so rigid to me in that hard chair. I, on the other hand, am more relaxed in this rocking chair. I want to feel more relaxed as I do now. I want to not worry. But you guys scare me. You always try to scare me. Why do you do that?

DR: PEARL: You ready to switch chairs?

ME Yes.

DR: PEARL: Go.

ME: Wow. It feels different over here. I feel more uptight!

DR: PEARL: Okay, speak. Respond. Respond to Nancy's question.

WHAT IFS: Well, I am here, we are here, to keep you on track.
To make sure you don't fuck up. WE don't trust you entirely.
We're concerned about you too. We don't want you to hope
for something and then be disappointed. I know. Even as we
talk, we realize we're a little rigid. But that's just the way we are.
We have our own purpose.

ME: I'm going to jump into the rocking chair now, Dr. Pearl.

DR. PEARL: Go!!

ME: (In rocking chair). I don't believe you. I don't think you
really do have a purpose. I think you are just trying to scare me.
I think you guys are the devil. I think you are my demons and
you are mean. And you are trying to fill me with fright. I don't
think you're very nice. I don't believe you have a purpose!

DR: PEARL: Good job. Back to the table. Respond!

WHAT IFS: Wow. Okay. Well, maybe our purpose is fear.
Maybe we're just fear. Maybe that's who we are. But I can tell
you're angry with us. Please don't hate us. We don't mean
harm. I know you think we're the devil, and maybe we are a
little bit. But maybe if you could just love us, we would soften.
If you could just love us, we would soften.

DR: PEARL: Rocking chair. Go!

ME: Hmm...I didn't realize you guys need love. Is that what keeps you so rigid? Are you just demons because you need love? Do demons just need love?

Dr. Self, I think I'm done. I think I've figured something out.

DR: PEARL: *Okay, come back to the couch. Let's integrate what you've found.*

ME: (back on couch) I think the "What ifs" are my demons. But deep down I think they don't really want to cause harm. And perhaps that's true of all demons. Maybe demons are just spirits that really need love. They need love so badly. And when they don't get it, they turn mean. And critical. And judgmental. And they try to scare us.

DR: PEARL: *So, what was that like for you? What did you learn about your own process?*

ME: Well, I noticed initially, when I was in the "What If" chair, my body was feeling rigid. But after she (ME) attacked me, it sunk in. I (the What Ifs) didn't want to be attacked. I (they) felt bad. I (they) wanted love. Then when I returned to the rocking chair, I realized that I was the stronger one in the relationship. And I had the power to actually help the What If's by loving them. Instead of fearing them, I could love them.

DR: PEARL: *You could love them....*

ME: So, I guess, rather than fear or hate the "What Ifs," I want to try being gentle with them. Hello, little What Ifs. It's me. I'm your friend. It's okay. I love you. Come sit up on the couch here with me, What Ifs. Sit up on the couch with me, Lenny, and Charlie. There's room for all of us. I have enough love in me for all of us.

DR: PEARL: *How are you feeling right now?*

ME Good. Integrated. I love Gestalt work!

DR: PEARL: I know. Me too!

ME: I think I'm done for the morning. I think I'm ready to go walk Lenny and Charlie.

DR: PEARL: Sounds like plan.

ME: Love you, self.

DR: PEARL: Love you back.

Later,

Thanks for listening everyone....

In Between Session Prayer:

Dear Lord,
Please help us with *"Vessel"* today. Please guide us in the recording. Please have everything turn out exactly as it should. Please be with us. Mom, you're here too...
Thank you,
Love,
Nancy

SESSION #25

....

Prayer.

I begin my session with Prayer. Pray before everything. Guide my thoughts. Guide my words. Guide my writing. Help me to be a vessel.

I turn on Jango and select the Beatles station and "Help" comes on. "When I was younger so much younger than today, I never needed anybody's help in anyway…" Thank you, Lord, that I'm older and wiser and have learned that help can be a beautiful thing. It connects me to everyone else. I am no longer alone or pretending to be self-sufficient. Life as Group Therapy. We all have things to learn from each other.

Happy Hanukkah, Everyone! "Hanukkah is a time of miracles," my friend Holly taught me when I was lonely and terribly afraid that life would never get better.

So, I look for miracles now…where are the miracles *this* Hanukkah?

Ah! Suddenly, I realize there is one right in front of me.

James.

He is my Hanukkah miracle.

We met during Hanukkah.

"Oh, are you Jewish?" he asked as he noticed the menorah in my apartment. "Yes." He thought it was cool. I thought it was cool that he was a pastor. That he was spiritual. We sat and talked for an hour in my apartment. "Are you capable of having a platonic relationship with a woman?" I asked him. "Yes."

I was interviewing potential roommates.

In hindsight, having to leave my job was the best thing that could have ever happened to me. For it gave me the push that I needed to look for a roommate. Yes, it would be helpful to have someone share the rent now. But even more important than the financial piece, was the loneliness piece. I didn't realize just how lonely I had been until I allowed myself to have a roommate. I'd fallen into this distorted thinking trap that I had to be self-reliant. That it wasn't okay for a 46-year-old woman to have a roommate.

And then, of course, I ended up getting the job at the State Hospital two hours away and I was going to start a month after James moved in. What to do now? And all my friends and support were in State College where my apartment was. What to do now?

But G-d has a way of leading us ... I was blessed to find Bonnie and her son out in Indiana, PA. She was a nurse. She was also a grown woman, over 50. She needed a roommate too!

So, for the next couple of years I lived in two places. Back and forth between Indiana, PA and State College, PA. I'd come home during the week to my new family in Indiana and then travel on the weekends to my family in State College. My family of roommates and friends.

Even when I was alone in either home, there was something so comforting about seeing someone else's "stuff" there. Knowing that someone else would be coming home at some point. That I wasn't alone. No one should ever live alone. That's my bias. I admit it. Okay, no one ever *has to* live alone.

And again, I believe that everything works out exactly as it should. For if James and I had not been forced to be "roommates only on the weekends," we would have never had the opportunity to test the relationship. To realize that we had become friends and were talking on the phone during the week even though we weren't living together. That we missed each other and looked forward to seeing each other. That we were slowly getting to know each other. That by the time we had our first kiss in February— "I'm glad we got that out of the way," he said---by that time we had a solid friendship.

So, James is my Hanukkah miracle.

I had said a prayer on the sunshine cake I had baked. I prayed to G-d ... "Please, Lord, send me someone to love me whom I can love ... I really hope it's James ... that is up to you though...."

Well it was, and it is. James. My Hanukkah Miracle.

DR. PEARL: Your Hanukkah Miracle. Nice story, Nance. I can hear the gratitude in your voice. I can see your smile as you rejoice...so what else would you like to talk about today?

ME: Well, I guess I would like to share with them about the recording, and talk with you about the What Ifs which I must say are much more subdued now. They are being treated with love.

DR. PEARL: Okay, what would you like to start with?

ME: I think I'll talk about the recording. Because it really was a "life as group therapy" moment for me.

DR: PEARL: Go on.

ME: Well, I was so nervous all morning, of course. What if someone doesn't show up? That was my fear tape. Need to have some theme to channel the anxiety into, right? But then as I was thinking and driving (and not paying attention!), I almost had a car accident. And in that moment, I became so grateful. Thank you, Lord, for sparing me from the accident. That I'M not the one who didn't show up!

So, I got there a few minutes before 11 … warmed up my voice on the piano. Tuned my guitar. Prayed in the bathroom. Nick showed up right at 11. Yay! He started plugging things together and we chatted. He talked about how he would record all the parts individually to get as much control as possible even though we were recording it live in a concert hall.

Yes, we could do a few takes. He had his own equipment. Yes, planning to do this after he graduates in the spring. Yes, Nick, that's right. I am a psychologist. Yes, I am planning to combine psychology with music—going into assisted living places, working with dementia. Oh, that's cool. Hey, I think your recording knowledge is cool, Nick. And you'll keep playing drums too? Yes … I know … health insurance. Scary thing these days.

Connecting.…

Noon was the set time for others to arrive. Gabby showed up next. Sent me a text to let me know she was on her way. (Thanks, Gabby for allaying my anxiety!) Now there are 3 in group therapy. We set things up. We warm up. We chat. We feel nervous and excited inside. We laugh.…

12:05 ... JT not here yet ... should I panic ... should I worry?
Should I send a message? ... NO! In he walks....

Now there are 4. The group has grown.

Four in group therapy today. I am not alone.

DR. PEARL: *So just in that moment, in that gathering of everyone at once, you felt good. You felt connected.*

ME: Yes, I and was excited about being connected. To others and within. I was excited that I'd somehow managed to bring people together to create music. And that I was an integrated me. I was the musical psychologist. I didn't have to separate those parts of myself. And JT even greeted my guitar and said, "How's Pearl doing today?" The feeling of being known. I exist.

And as we played a take, and then a few more because we weren't quite synchronized, and then another, because I'd messed up my guitar part, and then another to be sure, with each take, as we played and messed up, and played again, and felt it, and laughed, and joked "hey no one walks this world alone," and reflected how fun it was that we were doing this live together, I felt the song come to life. Did it sound perfect? No. But it was real. It was the experience of Vessel...of four people sharing some moments of life together.

DR. PEARL: *So, you brought your song to life.*

ME: Yes. WE brought the song to life....

DR. PEARL: *Okay, so now what?*

ME: So now I wait. I wait for Nick to get back to me with the re-mastering. I wait to hear if my voice sounded shitty or "bottomed out" as I fear because I was so worried about everything else pre-recording that I neglected to make sure my voice was in tip-top shape. I worry if it will be "good enough" to share and I wonder if I will still want to share an imperfect version if I should perceive it be "flawed" in some way ... I mean nothing can be perfect. But what's good enough?
So those are my What Ifs, I guess ... What If it's not "good enough?" But you know, even as I write this, I trust that everything will work out exactly as it should.

Some people don't believe that. Some people don't like the idea that "everything happens for a reason."

Yet I can honestly say that I have never had a seemingly "bad" experience that I haven't been able to look back on later and makes sense of, and then see the learning that occurred as a result of this experience.

Of course, when I'm "IN" it ... in the darkness, the fear, the pain, I can't see the future ... but when I remind myself that good will come from this eventually, it helps me in the moment. And even it's not true, it still helps to believe that.

DR. PEARL: *When you're in the darkness, fear, or pain, it helps to believe that good will come from it.*

ME: Yes.

DR: PEARL: *Okay, Nancy. Anything else you'd like to share today?*

ME: Yes. Love. The therapeutic factor of love. It heals everything. So, I would just like to send love out and wish everyone a Happy Hanukkah, a Merry almost-Christmas, a Happy almost-Kwanzaa, and Happy any-other-holiday-I-may-not-be-aware-of to all!

DR: PEARL: Sounds good. Happy Holidays, everyone!

ME: Happy Holidays, Everyone!

In-Between-Session-Reflection

You're right, Tom Petty. The Waiting IS quite hard.

I wait. Wait to hear back from Nick. It's break from school. It's holiday time. May not hear back about the recording until January. Who knows ... I don't. Acceptance. Of things as they are.

Best way to deal with waiting? Focus on other things. Talk to brother. Get update on my dad's move. Focus on finishing up Christmas shopping. Focus on piano. Focus on making a new Indian style chicken for dinner tonight. Focus on clients. Focus on being a vessel....

There. I feel better.

Later,

Love you,

Nancy

SESSION #26

···

It's 3:00 in the morning.

I'm awakened from a bad dream which I can't remember.

All I know is that I'm filled with mixed emotions of sadness and fear, that I'm still kind of "emotionally hungover" from fighting and making up with James last night and still confused about what I'm doing wrong and what he's doing wrong, still confused about what we're both doing right, confused, tangled up inside, wishing we were both perfect human beings, knowing that neither of us are or can be, wishing that I could feel the spiritual magic running through me at all times, knowing that I am human and prone to negative emotions, knowing the thing that I need to do when I feel this way is to write....

Write.

Because writing rights the wrongs, it keeps me from looking around for a target to blame my uncomfortable feelings on.

I see this a lot with clients too. Blame.

Kids blame their parents. Parents blame kids. Spouses blame each other.

We have feelings. Fears. Insecurities. Unmet needs. Yet-to-be-met dreams.

Or maybe we are/I am just tired, or I ate too many Christmas cookies or baklava, or my throat hurts, or the 12 degree weather and my lack of desire to walk the dogs in the cold has me feeling like Oscar the Grouch.

So many different factors to throw into the multiple regression equation to come up with the answer to the research question(s): "What is making me feel so shitty? What is making me act so shitty? Am I really acting so shitty or maybe just a little bit shitty?"

Hmmm… but yes, writing gets it all out of me and sorts it out. Cleans me out. A good emotional enema. Yes, I know that's gross, but it's true, Crying, taking a good shit, and writing … they all can be very helpful tools for releasing all the pent up stuff inside of us, whatever it is. And when it's out, I can take a step back and just laugh at myself.

And if I get it out in a healthy way, then I don't have to take it out on others. Or myself.

We/I have to move through the pain, not around it. Don't stuff it. With weed, alcohol, food, whatever your drug of choice is for internalizing your pain. Don't throw it out on whatever targets just happen to be surrounding you.

So "going through the pain" is a constant process in life. It's not a one-time thing.

I guess part of me wanted to believe that it was. Because I believe from my "N of 1" study of my own experience, that we have an opportunity for a "major life crisis" which at the time feels like a horrible thing, but once we go through it, and come out the other side, we emerge as a new, improved version of ourselves.

The dark night of the soul---going through the dark night of the soul was the best thing that ever happened to me in hindsight. Being terrified all the time. Afraid of everything. Hopeless. Chain smoking. Running from home to home of friends in Illinois searching for a feeling of safety. Every nerve exposed to everyone I met. Not being able to get off the weed. Not wanting to because I couldn't face reality—it was way too scary. Not knowing who I was, who I'd become. Longing for the 14-year old strong girl I had been at one time. Not knowing at the time that I would find her, and when I did, she would be an even better version of herself.

So here I am on the other side. On the other side of the dark night of the soul. And when I'm feeling irritable, ungrateful, angry, resentful, it helps to get on the bathroom floor and pray and thank G-d and remember that there was a time that I sat in T.G.I. Fridays eating lunch by myself and wishing I were dead. And then I can be grateful.

But the pain still comes. Because if it didn't, I wouldn't be human. Nobody has a monopoly on joy or pain. It is simply part of the human experience.

So, when the pain comes, I must move through it, just as I moved through my major life crisis.

So, I write....

See, I feel better already.

Now what? Do I write more? Do I continue to write about something else I've been wanting to share with you all or do I wait and table it for later?

DR. PEARL: *What do you want to do?*

ME: I want to drink some orange juice to soothe my throat. I want to read for a little bit and then fall back asleep next to James. I want to sleep for a few hours and then get up and go to the grocery store early morning when it's quiet and enjoy the exercise I can get just by prancing down the aisles as I shop for ingredients for the lentil soup I'm going to make for the New Year's Eve gathering.

DR. PEARL: Sounds like a plan. You're smiling. I can tell you're feeling better.

ME: Yes. Thank you, self. All will be well....

DR: PEARL: All will be well.

SESSION #27

....

2:00 in the morning. Awake again. Racing thoughts. Racing emotions. Fear. Sadness. Confusion. Where is my life going? What am I doing with my career? I'm lonely.

Maybe it's time to go back on the "other side" again. Find a therapist to help me sort it out. Perhaps. The last time I went to therapy for myself it was with Susan. She was awesome. She helped me work through my conflict of wanting to go back to school for music but feeling guilty about it. She helped me. I achieved my goal. But finding someone else, the right fit, is challenging. And having done my dissertation on "psychologists seeking help for themselves," I know the challenges and the fears. Confidentiality. Fear of credibility. What would others think? And yet here I put it all down in a book for you all, so what's to fear? Time. The effort it takes to find someone.

We'll see. I won't rule it out. If it gets bad enough, I will do the research and find the connection I need to help me through this patch. I do better in therapy for myself when I can go in clearly identifying the conflict. Which probably sounds strange because as therapists, part of our job is to help clients identify those underlying conflicts.

Perhaps it is an extension of a career conflict again. School is on break. I miss piano lessons. I have been practicing diligently but get frustrated and I don't have my "piano therapist" right now to bring my frustrations to. Perhaps this is the therapy I am needing and missing. And I'm feeling isolated in my work. Yes, I have lunch with a colleague here and there, but it's not the same as walking into a place and being surrounded by people.

I miss collegiality. But I'm looking forward to starting a Neuropsychology class at LVC in a couple of weeks because it will be a place I go to every week where I am one among a group of people—hooray-and I will be focusing my brain and learning something new and exciting that I will be applying to my work. With Dementia. With music. The integration.

We all need these things. Me too. Which is why I'm excited about the Neuropsychology class as well. I have a feeling that I will feel better in a couple of weeks. That I'm a little bit in limbo right now so I'm second guessing myself and my goals.

We'll see … trust the process, Nancy.

Thanks for listening.

Later,

Love,

Nancy

SESSION #28

I sit and I pray for guidance. G-d please guide my writing today.

The White Noise.

He tells me to write about the white noise. The noise in my head. The noise that I discovered could be tuned out by magical marijuana so I could think clearly, and creatively...until magical marijuana took over and made me psychotic, exorbitantly anxious, and unable to cope.

But aahh ... tuning out the white noise. The voices inside my head. We all have them. We prefer to pretend that voices are relegated only to those whom we label as "schizophrenic," but we know that we all have them. Thoughts...voices...whatever you want to call them. I remember one time one of the patients in the hospital asked me about this. "Dr. Nancy, when they talk about people hearing voices, don't you think they're just thoughts?"

What do you think?

Like everything else, it's probably a continuum. Internalized critical voices become thoughts. Or they take on a life of their own and we feel like others are there and present with us. Unresolved conflicts.

We try to tune them out, medicate them away. Problem is, they are still there. So instead, perhaps sometimes it is better to learn to live with them. To befriend them, like the "What Ifs," or to dialogue with them to resolve the conflict.

Like, this morning. The voices: "You suck at piano. Why even bother?" "No, try harder. Keep practicing. You're not practicing hard enough or long enough!" "No, be gentle on yourself, Nancy. I'm proud of you for trying. Don't give up."

One voice teases me. Another cracks the whip. Another is kind and nurturing.

I practice piano in half hour chunks. Two half hour chunks broken up by a dog walk. I go to a meeting. I pray during the meeting. I hear G-d say to me, "Nancy, one hour a day of piano is fine. Two hours may be too much for you right now with everything else on your plate. You are still making progress...."

Thank you, Lord. G-d answers my prayers.

Like last week when I was feeling lonely and craving collegiality, and I talked to G-d about it, and then the next morning, I get a group text message from one of the women with whom I share office space wondering if anyone's seen her mittens; and then three of us are texting back and forth about mittens and there's that feeling one gets with a clothing item that you love- that makes you feel good- and how helpless you feel when you can't find it. And so there I am connecting with colleagues through group texting about mittens, loss, fear-- and it's lighthearted and I'm smiling. And suddenly, I realize ... I am not alone. I am connected with colleagues even though I'm in "private" practice. Not terminally private. Hooray. Thank you, Lord.

Anyhow, back to the voices. The voices that spoke to me as I practiced piano.

So ... my little voices, my friends, I see you. I acknowledge you. I know you have the best intentions. Allow me to address each of you. I will start with you, Teaser.

Teaser, you are just afraid. You don't want me to make a fool of myself. You fear me wasting my time, being disappointed if I put in a lot of time on piano and don't see results. You are just afraid for me so you tease me. I get it. I understand, Teaser.

And now you, Whipcracker. Whipcracker, you just want to motivate me, I know. You don't want me to give up on something that you know is important to me so you go to the other extreme and push me really hard. You don't mean to be mean, I know. Your intentions are good.

And finally, Gentle One. Gentle One, thank you for being kind and gentle and encouraging me. You help these other two. We all work together.

So, I live with my voices. I don't suppress them or chemically banish them. No, I come to understand them and their purpose in my life.

Just like I learn to live with the darkness....

Live with the darkness....

The other day I had a client share that she sees herself as having "high functioning depression." That is, she can function in her daily life, yet somehow, the darkness is always kind-of-just-there ... lingering with her. Like a familiar friend.

The Chinese symbol of yin and yang informs us that even in the light, there is a tiny hole of darkness, and even in the darkness, there is a tiny hole of light. Both exist at once....

I guess I can view the tiny bit of darkness as a friend as well ("Hello darkness, my old friend...." Thank you, Simon and Garfunkel). It is there to remind me ... perhaps to humble me

. To let me know that even when I'm feeling joyous, it is important to remember that darkness exists as well and it will be felt again. Yet conversely, even when I am in the darkness, there is always a glimmer of light.

A glimmer of light ... hope ... no matter how small, it is there. Well, I guess I'm going to end here for now. There were a couple of other things I wanted to write about but Gentle One has told me that they can wait until another session. They will come up again if they are supposed to ... trust the process.

Thanks for listening,

Love,

Nancy

SESSION #29

....

FEAR OF DEATH.

ACTUAL DEATH.

I had a therapeutic breakthrough this week. I'm 52. She was 54 when she died. My mother. Only two more years.

Perhaps I subconsciously believe that my end is near as well and that I have to "get it all in" before time runs out.

Ringo Starr is currently singing on Jango: "Everybody has a whole lot of life to live … but you've got to sit back, oh, you gotta relax … love every breath you breathe…."

You're right, Ringo. I agree with you.

Still, I feel like I can't fully "relax" until I accomplish this goal. Until I share this book. Because it is my piece in the puzzle. My piece to contribute to the life puzzle. My child that I must give birth to and send on its way.

"*Luna Eclipse*" and "*Sunbird*." My songs are my children as well. And I am watching them grow up. As I was learning music theory at LVC, I decided to see if I could translate "*Luna Eclipse*" from guitar to piano. With my new music theory knowledge, I could adapt it to piano. Hooray! And now as I practice piano, I become more creative in how I play it. My child moves from basic block chords to jazzing around as its body and brain develop with time and learning. And then I discover, a part of my other child, "*Sunbird*," can come in and function as the bridge, the B section that I've been trying to discover for a few years. My children are working together and growing up together. Hmmm….

So, I play the new combination at my sister-in-law's Christmas party/family recital. I find new venues to share my children instead of keeping them locked up inside my piano room/office.

2018:

Will I have this "book" completed this year?

Will the song "*Vessel*" (which I patiently-but not so patiently-but definitely more patiently than in the past await to hear the mix) be ready and good enough to share with you all?

Will I have said everything I need to say in case it's my only book and I die at 54 like my mom?

Will I keep enjoying the moment as I've been doing lately and trust as John Lennon shares that "Life is what happens to you while you're busy making other plans?"

There's more I want to say and share and time is running out.

No, really, literally. Like my computer just told me it's going to do some kind of update at 8:27 and it's 8:17 now and I can't figure out how to stop it from doing the update that will shut off my computer!!

Hold on, Nancy. Maybe time isn't running out. Figuratively or literally. I'm going to take a pause, grab some coffee, and figure out if I can save this computer from shutting down in 10 minutes.

....

I DID IT! I figured out how to stop my computer from re-starting in 10 minutes….

Aaah….

Symbolism.

Perhaps I'm not going to die at 54. Perhaps there is more life for me?

So, do I slow down on my goals? Trust that there is time?

Yes and no. It's a combo meal. I slow down enough so that I don't give myself a heart attack and remember to enjoy the moments like just sitting on the couch last night with James and being grateful that G-d filled this lonely girl's heart with love and taking time out of my "busy, oh, so important morning" to make some Chili and take Lenny and Charlie for a good walk that brings them joy.

But I stay focused enough so that I'm striving toward something because "when you give up your dream you die" and there is a wonderful feeling one experiences when you are working towards a goal and it's something that scares you and excites you and then you actually achieve it, like the way I felt when I had my recital last year and I sang Italian arias and had people playing with me on songs I'd written.

It's 8:37 am. Have I gotten it all in? Have I said everything I wanted to say in this "session?"

No. There is more. But there is more time. I believe that. I say it. I speak it into being. G-d hears me.

"Go make some Chili," G-d tells me. Write more next time.... Thanks, G-d.

Thanks for listening, whoever's listening.

Later,

Love,

Nancy

SESSION #30

I get the email from Nick.

"Nancy, here is a rough version of your song. Let me know your thoughts...."

Here's a rough version of your song.

Here it is. My moment.

I don't have any headphones with me, so I find an empty private room in the library where I can go listen.

Quiet Study Room 3 at LVC.

I enter. I put my computer on the table.

I get down on my knees. *"Please, Lord. Let it sound good." "Please, Lord. Let it sound good."*

I sit at the table. I download the song. It takes a while. My patience is tested but I am patient.

This is the moment. I'm scared and excited. This is the moment. My song. Our song. Recorded. Here we go.

I hit that big, blue arrow with my finger. PLAY. Here we go...

I listen.

There's my guitar. There's my voice. I hear myself. I hear my emotion. I hear my guitar cracking but that's okay.

Okay, here comes Gabby. I hear her beautiful flute playing. She adds to my song. I'm not alone. We are together. It feels good.

I'm not alone.

I listen. I listen.

Here comes JT on the piano. There he is. I smile. I smile as he plays with emotion and I sing out my emotion at the same time. I am not alone in this venture. Now, it's the three of us. Together. No one walks this world alone.

I'm happy. And yet I'm also sad. I'm not terribly thrilled about the sound of my own voice. My guitar is good enough. I don't expect much from myself from guitar, just to be able to play the part I've written. Gabby sounds flawless on flute. JT sounds perfect on piano. And Nick did a masterful job with the mix.

But me. My voice. Do I sound dark? I want to sound happier. I want to sound lighter. I sound dark.

I try to remember how I felt the day I recorded it. I felt great. I felt it. It wasn't forced. I felt the connection with others. I felt the meaning.

So why do I not like the way I sound?

Perhaps I should check it out with others. Let James listen. Let JT listen. Let Gabby listen.

It always helps to check things out with others.

I will do that. I will trust the process. I will not be sad. I will be happy that I have taken a step in recording my song so that I can share it with all of you. Will you like it? Will you think my voice sounds bad? Will you judge me negatively like some have judged Grammy performances that I thought were wonderful? Is there objective perception? Perhaps not.

It is 6:00. I will eat at the LVC cafeteria before my Neuropsychology class at 6:30.

I will be grateful that I am not looking in the mirror wishing I were dead, contemplating ways to kill myself painlessly or praying for cancer so I can die.

No. I will be grateful that last night I sat on the couch with James and texted my brother and Jenn throughout the Grammys so that it were as if we were all watching together. I will be grateful that I'm not alone.

No one walks this world alone, Nance.

I know.

Later,

Love,

ME

......

It's later. It's the next day. Kind of the same session, though.

I played the recording of "*Vessel*" for James last night. I didn't tell him my thoughts before I played it but he could sense that I was not fully pleased.

He loved it. He guessed that I'd wished I'd perhaps sang it half a step up, but that it was fine.

I hadn't thought about that. Maybe that's all it was. That I wrote my own song a tad too low for my voice! Or maybe if I had been vocalizing more rather than worrying so much about the recording, I would have hit the low notes just fine.

Does it really matter, though? I mean, does my voice have to be "perfect?" Isn't this song, this book, about my own flawed humanness? Isn't it about the light and darkness, the high and low that co-exist, even in my song?

James and I talked about it. It wouldn't make sense to go to all the trouble of re-recording it. Especially when others had put their time and hard work into it. It's not just about me and my voice. It's about WE.

It's about WE.

Off to see clients.... 😊

SESSION #31

....

"When I see you dying I'll know my end is also near."

My end is also near. Or is it? This "book" is nearing its end. Or is it?

I mean there really is no "end" to the book. It is just a piece of my journey. A sample of my journey.

There is more. There will be more. But this is the snapshot I want to share with you all for now.

That I've been through the dark night of the soul. That I know we're all connected. That we all wrestle with the Givens of Existence. That we all need to heal our wounds and to be our authentic selves and to follow our dreams. That love, and creativity, and spirituality can heal us and pull us through.

So when will I "end" this book?

DR. PEARL: Trust the process, Nancy. You'll know. Just like when you write a song. You intuitively know how to "end" it. You'll know....

ME: Yes, I'll know. I'll know. I'm not there yet. Just like the folks in the assisted living situation are not there yet.

Some of them may want to be. They might be withdrawing from life, waiting to be transformed. Unnatural dementia...the brain is withdrawing ... the body is still here. Yet, as my friend, Howie, observes, folks with dementia can be the most spiritual. They've cleared a space in losing themselves which opens them up to be filled spiritually. They are crossing over into the spiritual plane.

I do that sometimes myself. Sometimes I feel like I just want to live in the spiritual world. And I can make myself nuts when I start to think too much about how "none of this is real..."

So, then I must ground myself here in the world. Structure, connection, purposeful activity, new learning, new goals, challenges, and adventures....

Like starting a Music Theory Cognitive Stimulation group this week.

(Yay! It's happening. My psychologist-musician identity. I am integrating!)

I was so nervous at first, of course. Just driving there ... my friends, the "What Ifs," were with me. I gave them some love and reminded them to trust the process.

And so it began....

"I can't hear. I can't hear" kept repeating H. I gave her hugs and she smiled and by the end of the group I'd figured out a way to communicate the music theory lesson with her even though she couldn't hear.

"I can't see," N kept telling me. Yet, somehow, we got her to write the letter "B" for Bass and "T" for treble on her paper.

"It's never too late to learn something new" reflected D who recalled that she sang Alto in school.

By the end of the first group, they had learned that Bass was low, and Treble was high.

They could learn. They had fun. We had fun. My heart filled with joy and love. I'm excited for the next group!

When I see you dying, I'll know my end is also near.

We're all dying. Perhaps they are closer to death than I am? Of course, they think about it.

My father thinks about it. He watches all his contemporaries crossing over. He says he doesn't believe in an afterlife, but every now and then he says something that leads me to believe he secretly does.

I feel blessed that I got to heal all my resentments, "things-I-blamed-my-father-for" while he is still here in the material world.

I feel blessed that my mother has gone with me through the "Luna Eclipse" as I worked through my conflict of the "parts-of-her-I-wanted-to-keep-and-the-parts-of-her-I-needed-to-heal" and we are now working together on our musical journey.

Perhaps if I believe "for" my father, then somehow when he does cross over, I will still be able to feel his presence as I feel my mother's presence.

We'll see....

Well, I guess that's all for now. I'm going to eat some lunch, then practice piano.

I'm grateful that I get to be a psychologist/musician today. I'm grateful that I have plans with friends tonight. I'm grateful for every lesson I learn.

Thanks for listening.

Later,

Love,

Nancy

SESSION #32

···

STEP 1: Read over notes from last session(s).
STEP 2: Read over notes sent to self through e-mails.
STEP 3: Get on my knees and pray for guidance....

And here I am. Voila!

Good morning, Dr. Pearl. It's good to see you again today. It has been a while...

DR: PEARL: *Indeed, it has. How was your trip to Florida?*

ME: Nice. Everything it was supposed to be. Sun, beach, warmth, connection with James, laughter with my brother, a couple of conflicts here and there for some drama and learning, stress, frustration, joy, walking on the beach, Chocolate Mousse Pie, pepperoni pizza at the Phillies Spring Training game, anxiety at the airport, a safe landing, and home to see to the dogs ... ta da!

DR. PEARL: *Ta da!*

ME: Anyhow, it's good to be back here in front of the computer. I need to write. Been too long. I'm a little nervous though. Because I'm really not sure what I'm going to talk about today.

DR: PEARL: *What do you want to talk about?*

ME: Well, I have a page full of notes. And I know I can't "get it all in," just like I can't get everything on my "to do list" all in, just like I can't get all the life goals in. There is only finite time. I guess that's why I decided to start with writing today. If there is only so much time, start with what matters most. And right now, that is writing. Cleaning can wait. Piano can be later this afternoon. But for me, right now, writing comes first.

DR. PEARL: Writing comes first.

ME: So maybe that's what I want to talk about. What comes first for me. Because it's different for all of us. On any given day. What's jumping out at me from my list is my mother. Talking with my mother. I'd like to bring her into session today.

DR. PEARL: Okay, we can bring your mother into session today.

ME: Can I go get a cup of coffee first?

DR. PEARL: Yes, I'll wait....

ME: Thanks. Be right back..
....
....
....

Okay, got my coffee. I'm ready!

DR. PEARL: Okay. How would you like to do this? Would it help you to move around the room?

ME: Yes. I think I'll put myself in the rocking chair and put my mom at the table.

DR. PEARL: Okay, who would you like to start with? You or your mom?

ME: Well, since I'm already sitting at the table, how about I start with my mom?

DR. PEARL: Your choice.

ME: Okay. Let me just switch chairs to get a different perspective.

(I switch chairs)

PEARL: Hello, mamala. Look at you. You're all grown up. Thanks for bringing me in today. Thanks for talking about me.

Off to the rocking chair!

ME: Hi mommy. It's good to see you! And "accidentally," I've seated you right under your portrait. So, I can really see you. You look so beautiful in that portrait. You were so beautiful. And troubled. Crying in the bathroom. So many dreams unfulfilled. You transferred them on to me as parents do. I want to fulfill them for you. I want to heal your wounds for you, mom. I just don't know if I can do it all.

Switch!

PEARL: I don't expect you to do it all, mamala. I know you can't do it all. I couldn't either. I made mistakes. I tried to do too much. I placed my value on how much I could accomplish in a day. I envied those who had more than me rather than being grateful for what I had.

Switch! (You get the idea....)

ME: Yes, but you were also wonderful. You inspired so many people, mom. You were always encouraging others. You played the piano and laughed and made everything fun. I was a teenage bitch. I was always angry. I never understood the things you were trying to teach me. I never emptied the dishwasher. Can you believe that I love emptying the dishwasher now? I learned a lot from you, mom.

PEARL: I learned a lot from you too, Nancy. I'm still learning from you. I know you want to slow down. I know you're feeling pressure to accomplish so many things right now. And maybe I put some of that on you. Really, honey, I just want you to be happy. I'm so glad you found James. I was hoping you would. He really loves you. And your new extended family is wonderful too. As much as you think you don't "fit" sometimes, you really do fit. I see that. You have your place there. You've always felt like a weird outsider. And some of that may be my fault as well because I always wanted you to be more like me and want the things that I wanted. But I see you making your way in the world. And finding your place. And that is what matters. That you are happy and loved. I'm having fun watching you.

ME: Thank you, mommy. That means a lot to me. And just your giving me permission to lighten up a little bit helps too. And giving me permission to trust what I need to do in terms of priorities. It helps me to breathe easier. So, thank you...

Still, though, I want to keep including you. You sacrificed so much for me, mom. You always wanted to make sure I could experience whatever it was I wanted to experience. Yes, you forced me to experience some things I had no interest in as well but that's what parents do. I get it. Anyhow, even though deep down I'm more of an introvert who would like to just sit here and write or cloister myself up and write music that no one will hear, I want to get out there and share because not only does it make you happy, but as you have shown me, it helps others as well.

And it helps me too. Like when I was lying on my back for two weeks in the hospital after my scoliosis operation and you wheeled me up to the ward of children with terminal cancer and you played the piano while I sang. You taught me such a lesson I'll never forget.

Not only did you teach me about gratitude by helping me see that no matter what you're going through, someone is going through something harder, but you taught me how to get out of myself by helping others, and you taught me that music can bring joy to others and lift others, that it's not just mine to keep locked up in my bedroom.

PEARL: Well, I'm happy that had an impact on you. I am proud of you, mamala. You have my permission to follow your heart wherever it takes you. I trust you. I'll follow you now. Just let me interject here and there and offer an idea. I still may have some ideas. I still have some wisdom to bestow.

ME: I know you do, mommy. Believe me, I do. I tune in and listen for your voice. Your voice and G-d's voice. Those are the ones that guide me. And perhaps that quiet little voice inside me that is not quite yours, not quite G-d's, but the little spark, the little tiny, tiny spark that is my piece that I bring to the puzzle.

PEARL: The part that makes you a vessel among vessels.

ME: Yes! You get it, mommy.

PEARL: I get it, mamala. I love you. I love you so much.

ME: I love you too, mommy.

DR: PEARL: You're smiling. You're smiling such a big smile. And you look relaxed.

ME: I'm happy. And yes, I'm relaxed. She approves of me. She's proud of me. She's with me. And I have her permission to do … whatever.

Just like on her death bed: "Nancy, I fucked you up but I know you're going to unfuck yourself.…" She gives me permission again. To slow down. To do things my way. And at the same time gently asks me to stay open to some of her ideas because she still has wisdom to offer. And she takes responsibility for her mistakes. She teaches me. She learns from me. She's proud of me. I'm happy.

DR: PEARL: *I'm happy you're happy, Nancy…*

ME: Well, I guess that's all I want to write about today. I really just wanted to talk with her. First things first. I wrote. I feel better. I feel relaxed. Now, I will enjoy cleaning. Because I am relaxed inside. It's all out of me. I will go unpack my bag from Florida … do some laundry … empty the dishwasher.

DR: PEARL: *And empty the dishwasher.…*

ME: Thanks for listening, self.

DR: PEARL: *You're welcome. I love you.*

ME : I love you too.

SESSION #33

....

Good morning.

I'm aware of the date. It's March. It's 2018. One quarter into the year.

Will I make the supposed self-imposed deadline? Will I have this "book" ready to share by the end of the year and have my song ready? Will I at least have everything in the works to be published? Will I reach a goal before the end is near?

What if I don't? What if, with all the other things on my list of daily responsibilities, it cannot be met "in time?"

DR. PEARL: What if?

ME: **Fear of death** ... fear of running out of time before my dreams are achieved ... fear ... death ... fear ... death ... **DEATH!** So, I went to a beautiful funeral yesterday. I love funerals, for like my sister-in-law, Jeanie, noted "Every time I attend a funeral, I'm attending all the funerals I've ever been to...."

So, there I was standing in front of the grave watching James' grandmother's casket being lowered into the ground when suddenly out of nowhere, I burst into tears and it hit me that the last time I actually attended a *burial* and watched someone go into the ground was when I was 24 and it was my mom.

It was as if it was happening all over again. My mother was being lowered into the ground. And in the moment, I felt her spirit so strongly with me.

They were not tears of sadness. They were tears of spirit. Tears of feeling the interconnectedness of everyone and everything around me.

The pastor spoke of how funerals make us aware of our own mortality. My own mortality.

When I see you dying I'll know my end is also near.

I'm 52. I don't know what my timing is. Maybe I'll have another 30 or 40 years to get it all in. Maybe I won't.

But I have today.

When I was younger, I used to think of each day as a half-hour TV sit-com. You know, each day has a plot and a subplot, and in the end in all gets resolved.

Now, that I'm older, I think of each day more as a lifetime of its own. If this is my only day here, how do I want to live it?

Well, for one thing, I know I always want to do "the next right thing" as they say. So, when I'm ready to sit down and write and yet Lenny is butting his head against my leg and telling me **"Mommy, I need to go out for my morning walk,"** I know that the writing must wait, and I must attend to Lenny first.

At the same time, though, I must organize my life around my dreams, for only then do they have a chance of coming true. So, I talk about **"one song on the radio before I die,"** but really, honestly, it is also about "one book before I die," the book with the song, which I hope this will be.

What is in my control? What is not? What is part of G-d's plan? What is not?

I think I would like to talk with G-d this morning and have you all bear witness to that? Is that okay?

DR. PEARL: *Who are you asking, me or them?*

ME: Well, since I can't hear their voices, I guess I'm asking you?

DR. PEARL: *And I'm going to do what I always do as a therapist and redirect. What do YOU think?*

ME: I think it's fine. I check my motives: Is it helpful? Is it useful? Could it help me? Could it help others? Yes? Then it's fine.

DR. PEARL: *Go ahead, then.*

ME: Okay, first let me get a cup of coffee … and pee.…

…

ME: Okay, I'm back.

DR. PEARL: *You ready to talk with G-d?*

ME: Yes, I'm ready. I'm going to get down on my knees and pray first.…

Dear, G-d. It's easier for me to talk to you when I'm down on my knees. I feel more connected with you when I am humbled by being down on my knees on the floor, on a bathroom floor. The computer makes it a little harder, yet I want to try because I want to talk with you and have others bear witness.

Because I've been given a gift. You've shown me the way out of the darkness. You've taught me how to trust you.

I'm looking up now. I'm looking up and see you in the one lightbulb left in the chandelier where all the others have burnt out. I'm looking over now to the portrait of my mother where I feel you next to her and I know she is like one of Santa's elves now, working with you.

I know at some point I will be on the other side working with you as well.

I know that in the grand scheme of infinity, my work will continue and my job as an angel-elf will last forever, whereas my job as humanoid in the material world is only temporary.

Still, there are things I long to do in the material world for fear that there are things that I can only do while I am here in bodily form. There are things that I am supposed to do to play my part in making the world a better place.

We all have to play our parts in the healing of the world. Where my dreams intersect with your will and hope for the world, that is what I am supposed to do. I know this in my heart.

You've steered me away from the things that were purely self-indulgent and guided me to the things that have a purpose beyond just self.

So where am I headed? I want to know. I'd like to know. Am I going to publish this book? Who am I going to share it with? Is there a need? Will it help anyone?

What about music? What direction is that going to take? Am I going to keep working with people individually? Am I going to keep focusing on the music-theory-dementia-research even though the assisted living place had to discontinue the group because of budgetary concerns? Is this a sign that I am on the wrong path all together or do I reframe it as a "pilot study to see that it's working and maybe you've just taken it off my plate right now because I have too much coming up between now and the end of April like this presentation at the Pennsylvania Psychological Association which is really the live version of this book?"

Where am I headed? I want to know where it's going....

I want to speak for you right now and write "G-d:" like I do "Dr. Pearl:" and write what I hear you saying to me but I feel like it's disrespectful so instead I'm just going to share with my imaginary-or-not-so-imaginary audience what I hear you saying to me, G-d. The quiet voice I hear....

I hear you telling me to trust the process. To trust you, that you will guide me as you always do. That I don't have to have all the answers. That I don't have to know how it's all going to turn out.

That, like Mammaw, James' grandmother, who after 93 years of a faith-filled-life that was built on serving you and who just a couple of weeks ago, said "I'm done...I'm tired...I'm ready to go..." and laid down and went to sleep, and a week later crossed over, that I will know.

I will know when it's time. I will know when I'm done. I will know what's supposed to happen next as long as I keep turning it over to you and tuning in to you.

I'm sitting back and reflecting.

I'm breathing.

I'm listening.

I feel peaceful.

And now I'm smiling.

Thanks for listening...G-d, self, and anybody else.

Off I go into the rest of my day.

DR. PEARL: Have a good day. Love you.

ME: Love you, too.

SESSION #34

....

Catharsis.

The therapeutic factor of catharsis. Get it all out. Make sense of the emotions you get out.

Dr. Farber, we heard you were crying in group!

Of course, I was crying in group, you assholes. That's what you're supposed to do!

And so I cry now ... it's a good cry ... a cry of remembrance.

I watch "Party of Five" on Netflix, episodes I watched over 20 years ago but now with a different lens.

I watch as Bailey hits bottom with his alcoholism. I watched the progression. How a basically good guy went through his own progression until it reached a point where he could no longer control it. I watch as he weeps as he looks at his girlfriend in the hospital whom he has injured driving drunk and he is finally desperate enough to ask for help.

I remember my own gradual journey into chaos. I remember how a good girl in pain found a way to cope with her pain that seemed harmless at first, until it took over, gradually, and though she kept trying to control it, she could not. I cry as I recall looking at myself in the mirror after throwing up soup that I'd filled with marijuana hoping for some kind of relief when it was no longer working, looking at my haggard, tired sick face in the mirror and crying "What the hell happened to you? What the hell happened to you?!"

I cry now with tears dripping down on my computer keyboard as I recall the sadness, the desperation, the hopelessness I felt.

I sit back. I take a breath. I look around this apartment, at the portrait of my mother, at my guitar, at Lenny, and at the Christmas cards still on the wall ... I smile.

I am still in disbelief.

That I made it. That I made it out of the hole when I thought I never would.

I start to cry again as I recall sitting in Marianne's house, chain smoking, not being able to sleep, riddled with anxiety and wondering about taking all the Xanax and washing them down with a bottle of something...

I breathe a deep breath of relief as I recall sitting in my cousin Scotty's house, researching on the computer which Walmart stores in Florida sold bullets and guns and contemplating driving down to Florida, making a purchase, visiting my friend, Ina, getting high so I would be numb, and ending it.

I take another deep breath as I recall walking along the side of the road in Portland, Oregon, needing a break from the rehab which I was not ready for, walking along thinking what it would be like to just somehow fall into the traffic, wishing I could make the pain and fear and loneliness go away and not knowing how to do it and returning to the rehab and told that I was on "suicide watch."

Suicide watch.

I smile. I take a deep breath...for now I am the opposite of suicidal.

I now know the secret to life.

I know that we are all connected and I am NEVER alone. I know that every moment of pain passes. I know that at any moment, whatever I am feeling, millions of others are feeling the very same thing at the very same moment.

I smile as I think about what I've been through and the meaning of it.

The-psychologist-who-has-been-on-the-other-side (haven't we all?)

I smile as I think about taking a break and walking my Lenny and Charlie and listening to some Gershwin before I go back to working on my presentation for the Pennsylvania Psychological Association.

I smile as I think about how wonderful it feels to take good care of one's self and how later this afternoon I'm going to go join the indoor pool (meeting the goal I set of doing this by 3/18) and I'm going to swim laps—something I learned to do in summer camp when I was 12!

I smile as I think about how great it is to be able to set goals and reach them.

I smile as I think about going this evening with James to see a high school production of a musical.

I smile as I think about my new official niece and nephew because Becca and Nathan adopted them yesterday and I wonder if maybe one day I too will be a foster parent and/or adopt a child....?

I smile as I realize how much of the next chapter is unknown and I am open to enjoying the book of my life as it unfolds.

Happy St. Patricks' Day, everyone.

I'm wearing green. My favorite color. Green is for Growth.

Thanks for listening.

Later,

Love,

Nancy O'Nancy

SESSION #35

······································

FEAR OF DEATH

Not metaphorical death. Actual death. Not mine. His. Lenny's.

Lenny wakes up on Sunday and he can't move. He can't move and he won't eat. He shits on the floor. *That's okay, Lenny.* He tries to hold in his pee because he wants to be a good boy and not disappoint.

We go to the vet yesterday. We sit for 3 hours as they run every test possible and take X-rays…no obvious signs of cancer…the vet tells me she had hoped it would be positive for Lyme disease because we can treat that. **"Does he recognize you?"** she asks.

Good question.

I think he recognizes me.

An angel showed up—Randy, the handyman, who helped me carry Lenny into the car as Lenny pooped all over himself. **(Mom, do you have to tell them about this?** Sorry, Lenny).

Yes, he recognizes me. For as we sat yesterday after we got home, and I talked to him for an hour recalling all our happy memories out loud, he rested his head on my knee … he knows me.

Lenny and I talked about heaven and how when it is time for him to go he will meet his grandmother Pearl, and his doggie parents as well and he will have new legs and a strong body and will be able to run around as much as he likes with no curfew and when he wants to be alone he can be alone because sometimes he just likes his quiet time. I asked him to just let me know when he's ready to go. I asked him to promise me that when he is on the other side and he senses that mommy needs to hear from him that he and G-d will get together and find a magical way of letting me know that he is with me.

Fear of death. Not mine. His. Tears flowing out of me all day as I struggle with not wanting to believe that his end may be coming. *When I see you dying, I'll know my end is also near.*

FEAR OF RESPONSIBILITY

Choices. I must make choices. The vet says the words. Suggests that I may want to *"put him down…"* She knows I'm not ready. Not yet. Quality of life for a dog? If he can't walk, what kind of quality of life will he have? She wonders. If he can't move, eventually he will have bedsores, she tells me.

No. I am not ready to give up hope. I am not ready to make a choice like that. Let's see. An infection it may be, she suggests. They pump him with antibiotics and painkillers. She suggests we look and see if there is any improvement in the next 48 hours.

What if there is not? What are my choices? Can't I just let him do what Mammaw did? Not eat. Not drink. Eventually he will die naturally. Can't I just let him be outside in the sun that is starting to come with spring and let him die naturally if it is indeed his time? Must I make a "choice" to "put him down?"

FEAR OF RESPONSIBILITY. I have choices. My choice now is to take it one day at a time. He ate his pills this morning as I stuffed them in doggie chews. No. No "real food" though, I tell the vet's assistant who calls to check on him. No. No water. He did drink up his own urine from the floor … confused … I know.

I choose to wait and see. He does not appear to be suffering. Just confused. And immobile. He tried to move. He tried to get up but couldn't. His spirit is still willing. That is where my Lenny is right now.

FEAR OF ISOLATION:

When I lose Lenny, will I lose a part of myself? Or will he always be with me? Like my mom. Perhaps after he leaves me physically, he will be with me even more strongly, spiritually, like she is?

FEAR OF MEANINGLESSNESS:
No fucking way! This dog has had such a meaningful life … bringing love and joy to everyone he meets.

I love you, Lenny.

Time to go take a deep breath and get ready for clients.

Thanks for listening.

Love,

Nancy

SESSION #36

....

The unspoken money trap we get into:

Fear of running out, of "not having enough...."

Subconsciously leads to fear of not having needs met leads to **FEAR OF DEATH**...or maybe even **FEAR OF ISOLATION**? Can't keep up with the Joneses---now alone? Probably can find a way to relate it to any of the ultimate concerns.

Still, "fear of economic insecurity will leave us." Note it does not say "economic insecurity will leave us," just the fear of it...learning to be okay with it...trusting that essential needs will be met. Bed to sleep in? Check. Food to eat? Check.

I clear the space.

I clear the space.

I clear the space.

Job opportunities come my way—contract for this, or for that ... so grateful that they present themselves, yet at the same time, aware that to accept them out of fear at this point in my journey is not where I am being guided. Feeling called to a different purpose ... one that comes out of my near-death life changing experience: *"You were saved for a reason. You better do something about it."*

Too much on my plate … overwhelmed and overcommitted … okay, it's a good lesson. Now that I see what it's like to have too much on my plate, I pull back. *How dare you say no??* There it is again. No, no, no … little voice of fear … I've got you, honey. *Fear of economic insecurity will leave us.*

So, I clear the space. I start to say, "No, thank you." I clear the space for the things that call me. And trust that even after new tires for "Slim Joe Blue" today who will be turning 100,000 miles (and I've never driven a car that long without crashing it!) and a wheelchair for Lenny, I will be okay.…

LENNY – my baby. I learn so much from him. He is so determined not to give up. He saw me getting ready to take Charlie for a walk yesterday and for the first time in days, said, **"Hey, I'd like to go too!"** He didn't care that he would walk 5 steps and then fall down and have to take a break. No, he did what he could. Determined. He's not giving up on life. Or walking.

So, I learn from Lenny. I won't give up either. *"When you give up your dream, you die,"* says Nick from Flashdance.

Okay, Nick. We're not giving up. **One song on the radio before I die.**

So, the recording is done. Volume levels tweaked. Re-mastered as they say. Thank you, Nick-not-the one-from-Flashdance! And I'm happy with it. Happy with the beauty of imperfection. With the beauty of my voice going flat on one note and my plucking the wrong guitar string on another.

Beauty in authenticity and my being an imperfect human being.

Just yesterday, a client of mine was feeling the darkness and the gloom and I asked him what little things brought him joy.

He reflected and then shared, "Finding beauty … in everything … *putting* beauty in everything, even in the things that most people would say are not beautiful … like walking up to a dumpster, looking at it and thinking, "Hey, this is beautiful."

I love this. Thank you, client. The learning always goes both ways. We learn from each other.

So … my Lenny and I are both transforming into a new way of being. Tomorrow night we will go check out a wheelchair that we may buy from my friend, Janis, who no longer needs hers as her doggie has crossed over.

Today, I will say, "No, thank you" to an opportunity that I thought about accepting out of fear, and put my energy into working on what I feel called to do.…

So … it is now April. Happy April. It is the anniversary of the day Martin Luther King was assassinated. "I have a dream.…"

I have many dreams. And I won't achieve them all. But I will achieve some. **One song on the radio before I die.**

So when will this book end?

Intuitively, I know it's May. May will be a year since I began writing.

Will I have said everything I want to say? No.

Will I have said enough? Yes.

Will there be opportunities to say more? Perhaps.

Like I tell my clients as we are getting ready to terminate, and they have a hard time letting go, and I have a hard time letting go, "We have done a piece of work together."

Okay, not ready to terminate yet. Fear of letting go.

DR. SELF: But you don't have to let go. You can keep writing.

ME: I know that. And I will keep writing. I'm always writing. This is about writing therapy. This is how we work through things. It's just that I know at some point if I want to share this with them, I need to close up this particular "book." Of course, I'll continue writing on my own...how else would I figure things out....

DR. SELF: Aaah ... so as with therapy, you learn that the work continues. That you keep doing what you were doing even after we "terminate."

ME: Exactly.

DR. SELF: Good job, Nancy/Grace/Luna.

ME: Thank you, self.

Okay, time to go get ready for clients.

Thanks for listening.

Later,

Love,

Nancy 😊

SESSION #37

···

ANGER!!!!

NO!!!!!!!!

Oh, those exclamation points feel good. "Just say no," says Nancy Reagan. "Just say no," says Nancy Farber Kent.

Nooooooooooooo!!

Aaah ... that feels so good.

Anger. Release it. Anger at perceived demands put upon me. Anger at myself for the tendency to "people-please" and feel like I have to say yes when I want to say no. Anger at people who say, "I never get angry" because after 52 years as a psychologist and a human being, I know that's bullshit. Everyone feels everything. We may not act on it. And we work not to act on it. But we all feel EVERYTHING!!!

So ... I release my anger-but not on others-and not on myself. Stay away from homicide. Stay away from suicide. Stay away from blowing up at someone else (progress ...); stay away from self-destructive behavior (lots of progress).

Instead, channel the emotion into positive addictions---writing, music.

I remember back when I was writing my way through my addiction. Praying at every turn in my writing that this would be "the last joint I lit up," and it never was. I remember writing "Positive addictions ... they are coming."

If I write it into being, it happens! If I speak it into being, it happens. The "law of attraction" as they say in "The Secret." I take a deep breath. I feel better. The anger is diffusing. I write it away. I laugh. I am able to take a step back and know that on the other side of anger is just fear ... sweet little fear. My friend, fear, who worries for me.

FEAR: Nancy, I'm afraid for you. I'm afraid you won't be able to say "no" to things and you will keep trudging along in life settling for less than your heart's desire because of me.

ME: Now, now, little friend fear ... you need not worry. I will take you with me and protect you as we head into the unknown ... into uncharted territories. Listen, fear, remember when we drove to Alaska together when we were 28?

FEAR: Oh yeah, I remember! (laughing)

ME: Yes, you're laughing. Remember how freaked out you were as we were heading over the Goethals Bridge?

FEAR: Yes, I was the "What Ifs." What if something goes wrong? What if we can't find a place to sleep tonight? What if ... what if ... what if....

ME: Yes, and remember how quiet you got once we learned how to trust and follow our intuition? We had our trip all laid out with a Trip-Tik from AAA. But by Day 2 we didn't need the stupid TripTik anymore. We trusted ourselves. We always found a youth hostel or a campsite to stay in, and when all else failed, a Motel 6.

But the turning point was when we got to Buffalo, Wyoming and it was teeming rain. We couldn't camp, there was no youth hostel in sight, and all the motels were booked up because the bikers were traveling through on their way to the motorcycle rally in Sturgis, South Dakota.

We knocked on that one motel door and talked to the guy who explained to us why all the motels were full. And then he offered to rent us his "mother in law's camper" for 15 bucks. We had the best night. Huddled up in the cozy camper, listening to the teeming rain pattering down and reading his mother-in-law's magazines. Cozy and safe.

FEAR: Not a peep from me....

ME: No, you got really quiet as we went along on the trip.

...

DR. PEARL: You just got quiet too, Nancy. And you're smiling. What are you thinking?

ME: I'm thinking that my drive across the country was a microcosm for life. I made it to Alaska. I reached my goal ... yet how I got there, the process ... I could not have planned that or told you how it was going to go. And I remember too, that it's not just about the destination. It's about the journey. So, I must enjoy the journey. Enjoy the challenges. Enjoy the emotion du jour that comes my way and enjoy my creativity as I am guided intuitively as to how to address the emotion...like being guided to write today ... and now feeling calm.

DR. PEARL: Calm

ME: Calm.

DR. PEARL: Calm

ME: The way of emotion is through it, not around it. Through it, not around it.

DR. PEARL: Indeed. You know a thing or two. We know a thing or two.

ME: Yes, we do....

SESSION #38

....

Here I sit on my metaphoric Goethal's Bridge—the bridge that took me on the way out of New York as I headed out on my journey to Alaska—the What If's and the unknowns going through my head and feeling the anxiety in my body.

I feel the same anxiety now as I get ready to go to my presentation for the Pennsylvania Psychological Association. I sit here in my room at the Sheraton in Pittsburgh and think about the reality that in some way I will be "coming out." I will be making myself vulnerable. Yes, fellow psychologists, I was in a psychiatric hospital. I was suicidal. I was addicted. I was crazy.

Do you still accept me? Do I still have something to contribute? Is this my something to contribute?

I write. I take a deep breath. The anxiety subsides ever so slightly.

I am grateful that I am connected. That last night, I got phone calls/texts from Holly, Lauren, Matt, and my James. I am not alone. I am connected even when I am 4 hours from home. I am connected when I talk to the barista at the coffee stand this morning and she laughs because she had to restrain herself from yelling at me when I opened my orange juice bottle with my teeth; reminding herself that I wasn't her 11-year-old son. I laugh and tell her it would have been okay if she yelled at me, and I guess I'm lucky that I didn't break my teeth opening the orange juice that way. We share a moment. We are two human beings connected. I am not alone. I am never alone.

Okay, little anxiety. You are still here a bit. But that's okay. I know you mean well.

DR. PEARL: Can I help?

ME: Can you give me a magic pill to make the anxiety subside a bit?

DR. PEARL: Do you want a magic pill?

ME: No. I've had enough magic pills in my life, and I know where they take me. I want to do this naturally. Like when I drove to Alaska and the anxiety subsided.

DR. PEARL: So drive to Alaska. Go there. Bring to mind a place on your journey where you felt calm and peaceful.

ME: Hmmm ...... Wells, Nevada.

DR. PEARL: Tell them about Wells, Nevada.

ME: Wells, Nevada. There was nothing there. Nothing. Just a small motel in the middle of nowhere. Me, a motel room, and Wells, Nevada. And I was at peace.

DR. PEARL: Okay, you are now in Wells, Nevada. How do you feel?

ME: Calmer. My breathing is deeper. More open. I am in Wells, Nevada. Safe, secure, smiling with a little secret in my heart. Hmmm ... I think I'm just going to pretend I am in Wells, Nevada and keep this feeling with me as I go get ready.

DR. PEARL: Sounds good. Poof! It is not the Sheraton. It is a little motel room in Wells, Nevada.

ME: Cool! This is fun. Thanks for your help.

DR. PEARL: Anytime. I'm always here for you.

SESSION #39

....

Good morning, friends. It is the end of April. May is almost here. My birthday is almost here. Turning 53 soon. Hooray, I'm turning 53! There's more life.

I'm not sure where my writing therapy is going to take me today. And my consciousness has been raised about how I never really know what lies ahead.

I never really know what lies ahead. Like on the road to Alaska.

I never really know what lies ahead. Like with Lenny now living a new kind of life in which he can hop-a-long for about 10 steps and then needs to rest, but he still prefers that to a wheelchair because he values his independence.

I never really know what lies ahead. Like going to the pool to swim laps last Monday, and not knowing that while drying my hair in the locker room, I would gash my head on the old-fashioned dryer on the wall and end up in the emergency room praying as they stapled my head back together.

One never knows what lies ahead....

So, I sit here with seven staples in my head feeling grateful that I'm remembering how to follow my intuition as I did on the road to Alaska. Feeling grateful that the accomplishment junkie that I've become, perhaps in response to guilt and shame over having been a marijuana junkie, trusted her instincts yesterday and spent the day lying on the couch, reading, watching Netflix, and recharging her battery.

I am recharged.

After a crazy day of blood gushing from my head in the locker room and my first vain thought being "Oh no, this can't be happening. My hair's not done yet!" And my second fearful thought being, "Oh shit! Everything I've learned in neuropsychology. My life will be changed forever by a traumatic brain injury." And my third thought being, "How the hell am I going to drive myself to the emergency room with blood dripping down my face? I won't be able to see through the windshield."

But eventually, my intuition told me to grab my purse, go upstairs and have the staff call my husband. And their intuition told them to call the emergency medical personnel. And it ended up being a high blood pressured, yet fun, crazy adventure in which I could get some perspective and gratitude and even enjoy the weird observation that James and I got to spend the afternoon together in the emergency room. It ended up being another life lesson in which I am reminded that I need to slow down and enjoy the moments with people I love because I am/we are going to die one day.

I am recharged.

After sitting in front of my computer for 12 hours finishing my neuropsychology paper about research on music, its effect on the brain, and the possibilities in treating dementia, and realizing that although I was exhausted, I was completely engaged, excited and enjoying the process of what I was doing, and when you're in that kind of zone, engaged in that kind of purposeful activity, **FEAR OF MEANINGLESSNESS** is kept at bay.

I am recharged.

After driving back from Pittsburgh, the site of where Alex in Flashdance decided to NOT *give up her dream before she dies*, and where Nancy Farber Kent got to play her song that she wrote when she was 26 years old--a time when she thought she was the only one who experienced darkness-- and then talk about existential theory and review the research that shows that existential well-being is negatively correlated with depression and suicidal ideation, and act out her own suicidal ideation story for other psychologists and be accepted by her peers, and then sit with the other psychologists in a circle and listen as they tell their suicidal ideation stories....

And then I know.

I know that I am on the right path, and everything that I have gone through, being the "psychologist on the other side" has meaning and purpose. And I take a step back. And I see. That I am integrated. I am a scientist-musician-professor-psychologist-dogmother-wife-daughter-sister-aunt-friend-human being. I am integrated.

It feels good to be integrated.

Today I am going to the library. I am going to listen to a talk by an author. I am hopefully going to be inspired as I finish this book and allow myself to embrace another part of my identity. *Writer.* Writer with seven staples in her head. Writer.

Later,

Love,

Nancy ☺

SESSION #40

....

Good morning!

Today's session will take place in a coffee shop. Like the old days back at Jackson Avenue Coffee.

The old days. I'm conscious that it is May and this book is coming to end an end. I've made a decision.

May 30th. I've scheduled my last session (for this book, anyway) for May 30th.

DR. PEARL: Sounds good, Nancy. May 30th it is. Do you want to tell them why you've scheduled our "last session" for this date?

ME: Sure. May 30th is my mother's birthday. So, since my mother and I are journeying together on this goal of "**one song on the radio before I die**," and my intuition had told me to end the book in May, it seems fitting to end it on her birthday, what would have been her 83rd birthday.

I look to the numbers. 83.

I long to find some spiritual significance in the numbers. Perhaps there is. Perhaps there is not. Perhaps I get to choose to perceive significance. Numerology tells me that we add up the 8 and the 3 and get to 11. We don't reduce the 11 because it is a "master number." It is the "most intuitive" of all numbers associated with faith. I CHOOSE to the see the positive meaning.

So, I will end this book on my mother's 83rd birthday.
Although, you and I both know there is never really, an "end."
Things don't get wrapped up in nice little packages with bows
with a "ta-da!" that symbols "THE END."

And yet they do. We have cadences. The music stops. And
then a new phrase begins. And then a new phase begins.

We have codas with "alternate endings," ones we didn't expect,
ones we choose to create.

Yes, I'm mixing metaphors but I don't care. This is who I am.
I'm a bunch of mixed metaphors.

And I'm rambling. Because I'm thinking about bringing up the
thing that I don't want to bring up in this session so I'm just
rambling and storytelling as clients often do until you, therapist-
self, challenge me on this. Until you ask me what's going on
with me right in this moment.

*DR. PEARL: Okay, Nancy. What's going on with you right in this
moment?*

ME: I'm thinking that I need to get home to Lenny. That I
need to be with him as much as I can right now.

James thinks that Lenny only has a few days to live. Lenny
stopped walking again last week. He stopped eating. He's still
drinking, though.

I've perused the internet to see what to expect. I know his end
is near.

Is it this week? Next week? I don't know.

Do I need to "put him down?" For now, no. He doesn't seem
like he's suffering. He still puts his head on my knee and
appreciates it when I stroke him and tell him how much I love
him and tell him to let me know if he wants me to do the
euthanasia thing because if he does, then I will do it.

He seems to be telling me not to for now. He seems to be telling me that just like with rejecting the wheelchair, he wants to die naturally, independently, at home.

My mother wanted to die at home but she ended up dying in the hospital. Perhaps she will get her wish through Lenny, who on some level, I always wondered if perhaps he is my mother re-incarnated because unlike most Labs, he feared going into the water to swim. And my mother had a terrible fear of water as well ... they both had eczema and itched and scratched like crazy as well!

So, Lenny. My baby.

I don't feel sad yet because I am in auto-pilot mode of just-be-there-to-comfort-Lenny. Change his bedding frequently so he doesn't have to sit in his own urine. Be "Nurse Nancy" like I was to my mother when she was dying. Sit with him and remember the great memories and remind him of what a wonderful dog he's been and how I know that G-d sent him my way to help me through the hardest chapter of my life.

Lenny. My baby.

What am I doing sitting in this coffee shop writing? There will be more time in the coffee shop later. There will be more coffee shops in other towns. There will be new chapters and new challenges.

Right now, though, for today, it's about Lenny.

Time to go be with my Lenny.

Thanks for listening.

Love,

Nancy

SESSION #41

....

As we get ready to "terminate" therapy, usually, we wean off sessions more. Sometimes we move to every other week. It varies though. And there is no one right way. In my case, with this book, however, it looks like it will be best for me to have more frequent sessions as I head up to May 30 which is approaching next week. That is what my intuition is telling me to do.

For here I sit with Lenny, who is lifting his head only on occasion now. His breathing seems more labored. He twitched a couple of times. Still drinking though.

Cancel my clients or not? That was the dilemma for today. Not wanting to let clients down. And of course, if I don't see clients, I don't get paid. But **FEAR OF ISOLATION** through disappointing others and **FEAR OF DEATH** through irrational fear of not having enough money are kept at bay today as I listen to the rain pour down and know that Lenny's time is limited and so I must spend every moment I can with my furry, baby boy.

Little Charlie has been barking his head off for the past two days. That seems to be his coping mechanism. Make a lot of noise. He knows what's going on. And I tell him that I'm proud of him for being kind and patient as we focus on Lenny. Soon it will be just Charlie. And me and James.

I am grateful that at a moment of loneliness yesterday, just when I was thinking that I wished Lenny's old friends in Illinois and his new family an hour away were here to come say goodbye, just as I thought that, I received a text from a friend right here in town. She lost her dog recently.

So, we texted back and forth all evening while James was down at his mother's, building a plain pine box for Lenny and digging a grave in his mom's yard, so that Lenny can have a proper Jewish funeral and be buried close to us.

I am grateful for friends who text me. I am grateful for James. Before I met James, and it was just me and Lenny, I said a prayer to G-d: "G-d, please don't take Lenny from me until you have sent someone for me. Please wait to take him from me so I am not alone."

And G-d honored that. He more than honored that. The day I met James when I was interviewing him to be my roommate, Lenny, who was then 90-something pounds, jumped up on to James' lap as if to say, "Mommy, this one! I pick this one for you." Thanks, Lenny. You chose well for mommy. G-d has given me lots of bonus time with Lenny. It's been six years since James came into my life. And 3 ½ years since little Charlie joined us.

It's never too late to find the love of your life. It's never too late to find new people and animals to fill up your heart. *It's never too late to follow your dreams.*

But if you miss your window of time to be with the ones you love before they cross over … well, even then, it's not too late because you can be with them in spirit. As I am everyday with my mom. As I will be with Lenny.

Still, for now, I choose to sit here all day with my Lenny. Will he die today? I don't know. Perhaps he will die tomorrow, in which case, I will have to cancel Book Club, which I'm hosting, and worry about if everyone in Book Club will still like me because I had to cancel or not worry because I'm human and things happen. Perhaps he will die Thursday or Friday. Perhaps he will die this weekend which would be perfect timing for us to then go bury him.

Perhaps he will have a resurgence and magically come back to life and be his old self.

Perhaps I don't know how it's going to go.

My mother spiritually influenced her own her death. In the Jewish tradition, one needs to be buried within a day of their passing. My mother said she wanted to die on a Saturday so that all her friends could come to the funeral on a Sunday. And wouldn't you know it that when the clock struck midnight at the end of a Friday in August of 1989, my mother crossed over. At that moment, as I took her necklace off and put it around my neck, I felt this sudden shock of energy as if half of her spirit went off into the air somewhere, and the other half went directly into me.

Thanks mom, for giving us a full Saturday to plan your funeral. Thanks, mom, for giving me your spirit so that you are always with me.

So, Lenny, here I sit with you, on the floor next to you, typing on my laptop as I wonder about what and when your moment will be.

Well, I think I've written enough for now. I feel better writing, knowing that it's not up to me. It's up to you and G-d, Lenny. You guys are working this out together.
So, what shall I do today? Shall I still do the other emails/calls/administrative tasks that were on my plate today?

I will prioritize. I will do 2 to 3 things on my "to do" list. And the rest of the time I will sit with you, Lenny. I will pick up my guitar and work on remembering the chords for a song I wrote for you many years ago. I will play you your song. I will show you some videos we made many years ago as well. That is what I will do today.

Thanks for listening.

Later,

Love,

Nancy (Lenny's mom)

SESSION #42

....

Session #42. 42. It's the answer to the meaning of life according to Douglas Adams.

"Lenny, yesterday my life was filled with rain. Lenny, you came along and helped to ease the pain.

Now my dark days are gone, and my day's looking bright

Cause you're here in the morning and to kiss me goodnight.

Lenny, ooh, ooh, ooh. I love you."

A number of years ago, I re-wrote the lyrics to "Sunny" by Bobby Hebb and played it around the house and at open mic at Jackson Avenue Coffee.

I haven't really been playing guitar that much lately because I've been focusing on piano.

But my mother-in-law, who came to visit and say goodbye to Lenny the other night, reminded me that Lenny knows me playing guitar. So, for him, I re-learned the chords, made some adjustments to the lyrics and started playing it over and over for him as a way of saying goodbye.

Perhaps it helped him?

I know it helped me. Expression. Creativity. Sing and write my way through pain.

It's been an intense, spiritual week. Feeling everything. It's good to feel everything and not numb out anymore.

I had to make decisions **– FEAR OF RESPONSIBILITY!** – Do I let Lenny die naturally? Do I have him euthanized? Do I fear that I will regret it if he is euthanized? Will he suffer if I don't euthanize him? How do I know it's really his time and he is not coming back?

G-d heard my fears and guides me. I schedule a Euthanasia for this coming Monday morning, and my vet was kind enough to agree to come to our home even though it will be Memorial Day.

I really did hope, though, that he would die naturally. Throughout the week I'd been texting/calling/emailing so many people who get it, and love me and Lenny, and are supportive and wise and tell me that any decision I make will be the right decision. Any decision I make is the right decision.

FEAR OF RESPONSIBILITY.

And with any decision, there is only so much that is actually in my control. G-d intervenes and miracles and mystical coincidences happen as well.

Like yesterday early evening, when Lenny was breathing so rapidly, and his eyes were open and looked strange, and I started freaking out and thinking, "Oh my G-d! He's suffering! He's suffering! I'm a terrible mother. I've allowed him to suffer!" and I called James who assured me it was Cheyne Stokes breathing and that it was a normal part of the dying process. I wanted to believe him but I was afraid -**FEAR OF RESPONSIBILITY**- Have I made my dog suffer?!!

And so just at that moment, I cried out, "G-d help me!!" and wouldn't you know, just a moment later, James walked in the door, followed by the little girls in the neighborhood who stopped by to say goodbye to Lenny. James assured me the breathing was normal.

Of course, I'd already called the vet, freaking out, inquiring if I could have him euthanized immediately, but it turned out not to be necessary.

So, after going out for a quick bite of Sushi-and taking note that I did not need to self-medicate with Saki, but could just move through the feelings and cope in a healthy manner, and being grateful for how far I'd come because now instead of Lenny barking at me in the garage in Illinois when I'm getting high and he doesn't approve, instead, I am fully present and able to be there for my baby in the last hours of his life—I returned home.

And made myself a bed on the floor next to Lenny.

And slept soundly next to him to the lullaby of his Cheyne Stokes breathing.

And I awoke.

And as I cleaned the fenced in patio of the apartment (the upgraded apartment model so that Lenny would have a place to hang outside), there was a knock at the door.

It was the little girls again. They wanted to see if Lenny was dead yet and say goodbye to him again.

I decided to play them the Lenny/Sunny song.

"Lenny, the time I know has come for you to go.
Lenny, I hope you know I'll always love you so.

You're my sweet little boy, and you're so full of love.
And I know you'll be watching me from Heaven above.

Lenny, ooh, ooh, ooh. I love you."

The girls smiled and sang along and then ran outside. I could hear them outside singing, "Lenny, ooh … I love you."

And just at that moment, Lenny gasped. And took his last breath.

The girls came running back and knocked on the door. Somehow, they knew that Lenny had passed. They brought their little cousin and they wanted him to hear the song too. So, I played it again. And they sang along.

They then decided that they, Charlie, and I should all go for a walk in the sun. So, we did. And I smiled. And I laughed as the little girls skipped with Charlie and rode their bicycles, and allowed me to follow their lead.

I don't believe in coincidences.

I believe that G-d decided to send the young, vibrant little girls, to whom everything is new and fresh to my home this morning to help me say goodbye to Lenny.

So here I sit in the coffee shop writing.

Here I sit thinking, "No, I'm in no rush to go home now." I came here actually to get away from home because it's only so long I can look at my dead dog, even though I cleaned him and covered him with ice so he doesn't smell too bad, while I wait for James to get home from delivering babies.

The cycle of life: James delivers babies as my baby leaves the world.
And today is actually Lenny's half birthday. 14 1/2. A good, long happy life.

I know. I *know*, just as I have experienced with my mother, that Lenny will be with me in spirit. And as my friend Trish noted, I may feel him even more strongly in spirit than I did in body. I know this has been true with my mother.

So, **FEAR OF ISOLATION**? Losing a part of myself now that Lenny is gone? No fucking way. Distance doesn't mean separation. Just as my friends and family may be in other towns and states and dimensions, I am always connected. To everyone. And everything. No one walks this world, alone, Nance. No one!

Well, I guess that's all for now.

Tomorrow, my baby boy's body will go into the ground.

But his spirit will go...who knows? Probably lots of places.

Hopefully, some of it has already gone into me.

Thanks for listening.

Later,

Love,

Nancy

SESSION #43

So here I am. May 30. My mother's birthday.

Today is our last session. So, what do I want to say in this last session?

I'd like to begin with an excerpt from a poem I wrote when I was in the sixth grade:

In a deep dark hole, there is no one but me.

I have no friends, because I'm lonely as can be.

When I turn around, there is no one to see.

The only voice I hear, is the one that belongs to me....

My mother loved my "loneliness poem" and it also frightened her. She was afraid I would always feel this way. She asked if she could contribute a verse:

If only I could leave my world of loneliness,

And somehow rise above.

Then perhaps I could be one of the lucky ones,

And find someone to love.

Perhaps then, in some way, my mother and I have always been co-writing songs. Though she wasn't here physically, when I wrote *"Vessel,"* she was with me spiritually, and continues to be.

Lenny is with me in spirit now as well.

I feel strengthened by the angels that accompany me on my journey. I feel strengthened by knowing that all of you are here with me as well. I feel strengthened by having gone through the dark night of the soul, which allowed me to be vulnerable and forced me to connect authentically with other human beings. It put an end to the myth that I believed—that I was different, or less than, or more than, or more screwed up than others. Nah! We're all crazy!

It felt good to say to a new client yesterday, "Just so you know … suicidal thoughts are normal. I've been there too, in the dark place." It felt good to know that this gave him hope.

So … **one song on the radio before I die.** Have I met my goal? Is it all wrapped up in a nice little ending?

Here's the answer—yes, no, maybe, yes.

You see, what I've realized is that the "radio" is a medium. A vessel. Like me. Like you. My songs are already being shared— with my friends and family, at LVC, at open mics, at church. They are being shared with the little girls who come to comfort me and Lenny as he crosses over. My song is shared when I play the guitar and sing at Lenny's funeral on Sunday. My song goes out into the universe.

If you have read this book, then perhaps you will have connected to the link and heard my song. My song is shared. I exist. Meaning. Connection.

DR. PEARL: Yes, but the radio. It's not on the radio yet, right? How do you feel about that? What do you think about that? And what are you smiling about?

ME: You know why I'm smiling. If I speak it to being, it's real. It exists. It will happen. If I write it into being, it will happen. *"When you give up your dream, you die."* Says Nick from Flashdance.

Well, guess what? I'm still alive. It will happen....

DR. PEARL: It will happen.

ME: It will happen.

Dr. PEARL: Anything else you want to say before we say goodbye...for now?

ME: Happy 83rd birthday, mom. I love you!

And to everyone else, remember, whatever you are feeling, or thinking, at any given moment, millions of other people are feeling and thinking the exact same things at any given moment. You're not crazy. You're human. We are all connected. No one walks this world alone....

Thanks for listening,

Later,

Love,

Nancy ☺

VESSEL

(song lyrics)

People been talkin' 'bout me. They say I'm crazy.
People talk about me. Say I must be mad.
People talk about me. But they don't know me.
Oh, but they know me. I'm the part that makes them sad.

No one walks this world alone. No one walks this, no one
walks this, walks this world alone.
No one walks this world alone. No one walks this, no one
walks this world alone.

So, come on all my brothers, all my sisters, all my mothers.
Come on all my fathers. Work your pain out fine.
Come along my journey. For it's your journey.
I will be your vessel. You can be mine.

No one walks this world alone. No one walks this, no one
walks this, walks this world alone.
No one walks this world alone. No one walks this, no one
walks this world alone.

So, when I see you walkin,' well that's me walkin'.
When I hear you talkin,' it's my own words that I hear.
When you see me dancin,' well that's you dancin'.
When I see you dyin,' I'll know my end is also near.

No one walks this world alone. No one walks this, no one
walks this, walks this world alone.
No one walks this world alone. No one walks this, no one
walks this world alone.

To listen to "Vessel" visit the following link

www.soundcloud.com/user-770880052

Or scan the following QR code

REFERENCES

Adams, D. (1979). *The hitchhiker's guide to the galaxy.* London: Pan Books.

Bateson, M. C. (1989). *Composing a life.* New York: Grove Press.

Bearde, C., Blye, A., Arnott, B., Burditt, G., Hahn, P., Johnson, C., Wayne, P. Einstein, B., Martin, S. Mulligan, J., Brown, E. Hanrahan, J. (Writers). & Fisher, A. (Director). (1971-1974). The Sonny and Cher comedy hour. [Television series]. In Bearde, C., Blye, A. & Blye, G. (Producers). Hollywood, CA: CBS Television.

Bernstein, L. (1957). West side story (melodies). [Recorded by Stuttgart Radio Symphony Orchestra]. On *American portraits: West side story and other masterpieces.* [CD]. Santa Monica, CA: Delta Music, Inc. (1995).

Bernstein, L. (Composer), & Sondheim, S. (Lyricist). (1957, 1958, 1959). Choral selection from West Side Story. [sheet music arranged for mixed (S.A.T.B.) voices by W. Stickles]. New York: G. Schirmer, Inc. & Chappell & Co., Inc.

Byrne, R. (2006). *The secret.* New York: Atria Books/Beyond Word Capra, A. (Producer & Director). (1946). *It's a wonderful life.* [Motion Picture]. United States: RKO Radio Pictures.

Carmichael, H. (Composer) & Mercer, J. (Lyricist). (1941). Skylark. [Lead Sheet]. Retrieved from https://irealpro.com.

Clivillés, R. & William, F. B. (1990). Gonna make you sweat (Everybody dance now). [Recorded by C + C Music Factory]. On *Gonna make you sweat* (CD). New York: Columbia.

Decoz, H. & Monte, T. (1994). *Numerology: key to your inner self.* New York: Penguin Group.

Dunford, M. & Thatcher, B. (1973.). Let it grow. [Recorded by Renaissance]. On *Ashes are burning.* (LP). Wembley, UK: De Lane Lea Studios.

Farber. N. K. (1999). *Counseling psychology doctoral students' help seeking behavior: Factors affecting willingness to seek help for psychological problems.* (Doctoral Dissertation). Retrieved from ProQuest Dissertations and Theses A & I (Order No. 9950362).

Farber, N.K. (2000). Trainees' attitudes toward seeking psychotherapy scale: Development and validation of a research instrument. *Psychotherapy: Theory, Research, Practice, Training.* 37(4):341–353.

Farber, N. K. (2010) *Vessel.* [Recorded by Farber Kent, N. with Giarratano, G & Tindall, J.] (MIDI). Annville: Lebanon Valley College. (2017).

Freud, S. (2018). *The ego and the id.* Mineola, NY: Dover Publications, Inc. Goldberg, N. (1986). *Writing down the bones: Freeing the writer within.* Boston: Shambhala.

Gottlieb, L. (Producer). & Ardolino, E. (Director). (1987). *Dirty dancing.* [Motion Picture]. United States: Great American Films Limited Partnership.

Hamachek, D. E. (1982). *Encounters with others: Interpersonal relationships and you.* Orlando, FL: Harcourt, Brace Jovanovich.

Hebb, B. (1966). Sunny. On *Sunny* [LP]. New York: Philips.

Hirsch, J.K., Nsamenang, S. A., Chang, E. C. & Kaslow, N. J. (2014). Spiritual well-being and depressive symptoms in female African American suicide attempters: Mediating effects optimism and pessimism. *Psychology of Religion and Spirituality, 6, 276-283.*

Keach, J. & Konrad, C. (Producers). & Mangold, J. (Director). (2005). *Walk the line.* [Motion Picture]. United States: Fox 2000 Pictures.

Keagy, K. (1983). Sister Christian. [Recorded by Night Ranger]. On *Midnight madness* [LP]. Universal City, CA: MCA.

King, M. L., Jr. (1963, August 28). *I have a dream.* Retrieved from https://www.archives.gov/files/press/exhibits/dream-speech.pdf.

Le Bon, S. Taylor, J. Taylor, R., Taylor, A. & Rhodes, N. (1982). Rio. [Recorded by Duran Duran]. On *Rio* (LP). London: EMI.

Lennon, J., & McCartney, P. (1966). And your bird can sing. [Recorded by The Beatles] On *Revolver* [LP]. London: EMI.

Lennon, J. & McCartney, P. (1965). Help! [Recorded by The Beatles]. On *Help!* [LP]. London: EMI Studios. Retrieved www.jango.com.

Lennon, J. (1980). Beautiful boy (darling boy). On *Double fantasy* [LP]. New York: Geffen.

Marco, J.H., Guillén, V. & Botella, C. (2017). The buffer role of meaning in life in hopelessness in women with borderline personality disorders. *Psychiatry Research, 247,* 120-124.

Marvin, N. (Producer). & Darabont, F. (Director). (1994). *The Shawshank redemption.* [Motion Picture]. United States: Castle Rock Entertainment.

Palmer, M. (1997). *Yin and yang: Understanding the philosophy of opposites and how to apply it to your everyday life.* London: Piatkus.

Papazian, R.A., & Galli, H. (Producers). & Sargent, J. (Director). (1989). *The Karen Carpenter story.* [Motion Picture]. United States: Columbia Broadcasting System.

Petty, T. (1981). The waiting. [Recorded by Tom Petty and The Heartbreakers]. On *Hard promises.* [LP].Van Nuys and Hollywood, CA: Backstreet Records.

Reagan, N. (1986, September 14). *Just say no.* Retrieved from http://www.cnn.com/SPECIALS/2004/reagan/stories /speech.archive/just.say.no.html

Simon, S. (1965). The sound of silence. [Recorded by Simon & Garfunkel]. On *Sounds of silence* [LP]. New York and Los Angeles: Columbia Records.

Simonds, P.K. (Writer), & Gordon,D. (Director). (1997). Hitting bottom [Television series episode]. In Keyser, C. & Lippman, A. (Producers), *Party of five.* Culver City, CA: Columbia Pictures Television.

Simpson, D., Bruckheimer, J., Jacobson, T., Obst, L.R., Guber, P., & Peters, J. (Producers) & Lyne, A. (Director). (1983). *Flashdance*. [Motion Picture]. United States: Polygram Filmed Entertainment; Simpson/Bruckheimer.

Starkey, R., Hudson, M. & Dudas, S. (2008). Give it a try. (Recorded by Ringo Starr). On *Liverpool 8* [MP3]. London, Los Angeles: Capitol.

Taliaferro, L.A., Rienzo, B.A., Pigg, R.M., Miller, M.D., and Dodd, V.J. (2009). Spiritual well-being and suicidal ideation among college students. *Journal of American College Health, 58,* 83-90.

W., Bill. (1976). *Alcoholics Anonymous: the story of how many thousands of men and women have recovered from alcoholism.* New York: Alcoholics Anonymous World Services.

Waller, F. (Composer) & Razaf, A. (Lyricist). (1929). Honeysuckle Rose. [Lead Sheet]. Retrieved from https://irealpro.com.

Wechsler, D. (1997) Wechsler adult intelligence scale: Third Edition (WAIS-III) [Assessment Instrument].

Yalom, I. D. (1980). *Existential Psychotherapy.* New York: Basic Books.

Yalom, I. D. (1995). *The Theory and Practice of Group Psychotherapy.* New York: Basic Books.

Yalom, I.D. & Josselson, R. (2013). Existential Psychotherapy. In Wedding, D. & Corsini, R.J. (Eds.), *Current Psychotherapies* (10th ed., pp. 265-297). Belmont, CA: Brooks/Cole.

AUTHOR BIO

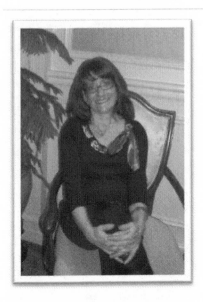

Nancy Farber Kent (Dr. Nancy K. Farber) is a licensed clinical psychologist, school counselor, and veteran professor of school, community, and clinical counseling who has worked in a variety of settings as both a psychotherapist and teacher. Dr. Farber currently works with clients in private practice and with older adults in assisted living facilities where she integrates music and cognitive stimulation therapy to improve memory in individuals with dementia.

Dr. Farber is also a published researcher who has written articles for peer-reviewed journals and presented both research and training workshops at national professional conferences including the American Psychological Association and the American School Counselor Association. She holds a B.A. in music from Lebanon Valley college, a Ph.D. in counseling psychology from Ball State University, an MS.Ed. in psychological services from the University of Pennsylvania, and a B.S. in communication arts from Cornell University.

For more information, please visit her website at **www.nancyfarberkent.com**